Dermatology:

Therapy

NORMAN LEVINE, MD

Clinical Professor of Medicine (Dermatology)
University of Arizona College of Medicine
Tucson, AZ

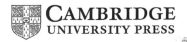

CAMBRIDGE
UNIVERSITY PRESS

CAMBRIDGE UNIVERSITY PRESS

Cambridge, New York, Melbourne, Madrid, Cape Town, Singapore, São Paulo, Delhi

Cambridge University Press
32 Avenue of the Americas, New York, NY 10013-2473, USA

www.cambridge.org
Information on this title: www.cambridge.org/9780521709330

First published 2007

Printed in the United States of America

A catalog record for this publication is available from the British Library.

Library of Congress Cataloging in Publication Data

Levine, Norman, 1945 Mar. 18-
Dermatology : diseases and therapy / Norman Levine.
    p. ; cm.
ISBN-13: 978-0-521-70933-0 (pbk.)
ISBN-10: 0-521-70933-4 (pbk.)
1. Dermatology – Handbooks, manuals, etc. 2.
Skin – Diseases – Handbooks, manuals, etc. I. Title.
[DNLM: 1. Skin Diseases – diagnosis – Handbooks. 2. Dermatologic
Agents – therapeutic use – Handbooks. 3. Skin
Diseases – therapy – Handbooks. WR 39 L665d 2007]
RL71.L57   2007
616.5 – dc22   2007016914

ISBN   978-0-521-70933-0 paperback

NOTICE

Because of the dynamic nature of medical practice and drug selection and dosage, users are advised that decisions regarding drug therapy must be based on the independent judgment of the clinician, changing information about a drug (e.g., as reflected in the literature and manufacturer's most current product information), and changing medical practices.

While great care has been taken to ensure the accuracy of the information presented, users are advised that the authors, editors, contributors, and publisher make no warranty, express or implied, with respect to, and are not responsible for, the currency, completeness, or accuracy of the information contained in this publication, nor for any errors, omissions, or the application of this information, nor for any consequences arising therefrom. Users are encouraged to confirm the information contained herein with other sources deemed authoritative. Ultimately, it is the responsibility of the treating physician, relying on experience and knowledge of the patient, to determine dosages and the best treatment for the patient. Therefore, the author(s), editors, contributors, and the publisher make no warranty, express or implied, and shall have no liability to any person or entity with regard to claims, loss, or damage caused, or alleged to be caused, directly or indirectly, by the use of information contained in this publication.

Further, the author(s), editors, contributors, and the publisher are not responsible for misuse of any of the information provided in this publication, for negligence by the user, or for any typographical errors.

Contents

Contents

Contents

PART TWO. THERAPY

Preface

The specific aims of this book are to give the practitioner an organized, condensed and practical approach to the patient with a skin problem. It includes the elements of diagnosis for hundreds of the most common cutaneous problems and provides recommendations for the management of these conditions. Also included are detailed descriptions of the most commonly used medications in dermatology today.

The book is written for the use of medical students, primary care practitioners, dermatology residents and practicing dermatologists.

Norman Levine

PART ONE

Diseases

ACANTHOSIS NIGRICANS

ALTERNATE DISEASE NAME
- None

HISTORY
- Gradual onset of asymptomatic areas of darkening & thickening of the skin
- History or family history of diabetes mellitus and/or insulin resistance, often in overweight pts
- Associated w/ endocrinopathies, such as hyperandrogenemia, or an autoimmune disease such as systemic lupus erythematosus, scleroderma, Sjögren syndrome or Hashimoto thyroiditis
- More common in people w/ darker skin pigmentation
- Rapidly evolving subset in adults associated w/ internal malignancy, particularly of the GI tract, where skin changes precede the malignancy diagnosis in 1/3 of cases

PHYSICAL EXAMINATION
- Symmetrical, hyperpigmented, velvety plaques, occurring in intertriginous areas, such as axillae & groin, on the nipples & on the neck
- Vulva is most commonly affected site in females in those who are hyperandrogenic & obese
- Skin tags in the vicinity of the plaques
- Physical findings identical for both the malignant & benign forms

DIFFERENTIAL DIAGNOSIS
- Becker nevus
- Confluent & reticulated papillomatosis of Gougerot & Carteaud
- Dowling-Degos disease
- Seborrheic keratosis
- Ichthyosis hystrix
- Linear epidermal nevus
- Parapsoriasis en plaque
- Pemphigus vegetans
- Pellagra

LABORATORY WORK-UP
- In adult-onset type, perform basic workup for underlying malignancy

■ In early-onset disease, particularly in obese pts, obtain serum insulin level & hemoglobin A1C

MANAGEMENT
■ Weight reduction in obese pts
■ Treat underlying malignancy, if present

SPECIFIC THERAPY
■ None

CAVEATS AND PITFALLS
■ Advise that pt is at risk for diabetes, even if there is no evidence at present.

ACNE KELOIDALIS

ALTERNATE DISEASE NAME
■ Acne keloidalis nuchae
■ Folliculitis keloidalis
■ Folliculitis keloidalis nuchae
■ Acne keloid

HISTORY
■ Occurs mainly in men of African descent, after puberty & before age 50
■ Begins as chronic folliculitis of posterior neck & occipital scalp
■ May be related to close shaving of hair and/or irritation from clothing

PHYSICAL EXAMINATION
■ Firm, dome-shaped, follicular papules on nape of neck and/or on occipital scalp
■ Papules coalesce into sclerotic plaques
■ Scarring alopecia & subcutaneous abscesses w/ draining sinuses later in the course

DIFFERENTIAL DIAGNOSIS
■ Folliculitis
■ Acne vulgaris
■ Perifolliculitis capitis
■ Nevus sebaceous

- Keloid
- Pediculosis capitis
- Squamous cell carcinoma
- Basal cell carcinoma

LABORATORY WORK-UP
- Skin biopsy if there is doubt of the diagnosis
- Culture for bacterial pathogens if there are pustules

MANAGEMENT
- Avoid potential trauma to neck & posterior scalp area, such as close-cropped hairstyles, tight-fitting hats
- Surgical excision
- Destruction by laser or liquid nitrogen cryotherapy
- Intralesional corticosteroids
- Systemic antibiotics for secondary bacterial infection or as anti-inflammatory agent

SPECIFIC THERAPY
- Tetracycline 500 mg PO BID; alternative is doxycycline 100 mg PO BID
- CO_2 laser vaporization followed by intralesional triamcinolone (5–10 mg/mL) or imiquimod 5% cream applied daily for 6–8 wks
- Triamcinolone (5–10 mg/mL) intralesional after softening the site w/ light liquid nitrogen cryotherapy
- Punch excision of individual papules
- Horizontal elliptical excision w/ or w/out primary closure

CAVEATS AND PITFALLS
- Once scarring has occurred, the skin does not return to normal.

ACNE VULGARIS

ALTERNATE DISEASE NAME
- Acne varus

HISTORY
- Peak incidence at puberty but may begin in first decade
- Women often have sustained activity until late 30's
- Severity may have genetic component
- Flares may occur in times of stress

PHYSICAL EXAMINATION
- Lesions in areas w/ abundant sebaceous follicles: face, back, upper chest wall
- Closed comedos (whitehead) & open comedos (blackhead)
- Inflammatory papules, pustules, nodules & cysts
- Draining sinuses
- Postinflammatory scars
- Hormonal component: flares w/ menses

DIFFERENTIAL DIAGNOSIS
- Acne aestivalis
- Rosacea
- Perioral dermatitis
- Folliculitis
- Acne medicamentosa
- Occupational acne
- Tropical acne
- Acne cosmetica
- Syndrome of Favre-Racouchot
- Flat warts
- Trichostasis spinulosa

LABORATORY WORK-UP
- None

MANAGEMENT
- Systemic antibiotics
- Topical antibiotics
- Topical retinoids
- Azelaic acid
- Isotretinoin
- Hormonal therapy
- Acne surgery

SPECIFIC THERAPY
- Tetracycline 250–500 mg PO BID
- Doxycycline 100 mg PO QD-BID
- Minocycline 50–100 mg PO BID
- Erythromycin 250–500 mg PO BID
- Topical 1% clindamycin solution, cream, gel or lotion applied BID; use w/ benzoyl peroxide to minimize drug resistance

- Topical 2% erythromycin solution, cream, lotion or gel applied BID; use w/ benzoyl peroxide to minimize drug resistance
- Benzoyl peroxide 5–10% gel or cream applied BID
- Tretinoin 0.025% cream applied HS; alternative is adapalene 0.1% gel applied HS
- Isotretinoin 1 mg/kg per day PO for 5 months; advise about strict contraception in women
- Spironolactone 100–200 mg PO per day in women only
- Oral contraceptives, particularly Desogen™ or Ortho Tri-Cyclen™
- Acne surgery, including comedo expression; incision & drainage of fluctuant cysts & abscesses; chemical peel; microdermabrasion; intralesional triamcinolone 2–4 mg/mL

CAVEATS AND PITFALLS
- Use isotretinoin only in severe scarring acne, unresponsive to other measures.
- Erythromycin has high incidence of early drug resistance.
- Doxycycline may produce sun sensitivity.
- Spironolactone may produce menstrual irregularity.
- Benzoyl peroxide may cause bleaching of clothes.

ACROANGIODERMATITIS

ALTERNATE DISEASE NAME
- Pseudo-Kaposi's sarcoma
- Mali disease

HISTORY
- Longstanding history of venous stasis (w/ bilateral involvement), arteriovenous shunt for hemodialysis, or arteriovenous malformation (w/ unilateral involvement)

PHYSICAL EXAMINATION
- Confluent, violaceous or brown-black papules & plaques over distal legs
- Occasional erosions, ulcerations and/or bleeding

DIFFERENTIAL DIAGNOSIS
- Kaposi's sarcoma
- Stasis dermatitis
- Contact dermatitis
- Lichen planus
- Lupus erythematosus
- Benign pigmented purpura
- Cutaneous vasculitis

LABORATORY WORK-UP
- Skin biopsy for routine light microscopy to rule out Kaposi's sarcoma
- Plethysmography, Doppler ultrasonography & oscillography to assess venous flow & to detect vascular malformations

MANAGEMENT
- Compression therapy
- Correct underlying venous disease

SPECIFIC THERAPY
- Unna boots
- Sequential compression device, 30–40 mm, applied 30–45 minutes per day
- Surgical excision of shunts if there is arteriovenous malformation

CAVEATS AND PITFALLS
- Goal of therapy is to reduce edema.

ACROCHORDON

ALTERNATE DISEASE NAME
- Skin tag
- Soft wart
- Fibroepithelial polyp

HISTORY
- Slow-growing asymptomatic lesions, most frequently on neck & axillae
- More common in obese pts
- May be associated w/ acanthosis nigricans

PHYSICAL EXAMINATION
- Round, soft, pedunculated papules, which are either flesh-colored or hyperpigmented
- May be tender or bleed when traumatized

DIFFERENTIAL DIAGNOSIS
- Wart
- Neurofibroma
- Seborrheic keratosis
- Melanocytic nevus
- Melanoma
- Fibroepithelioma of Pinkus
- Pseudosarcomatous polyp

LABORATORY WORK-UP
- None

MANAGEMENT
- Surgical removal

SPECIFIC THERAPY
- Scissors excision; use local anesthesia for broad-based lesions
- Liquid nitrogen cryotherapy; advise about post-procedure hypopigmentation
- Destruction by electrodesiccation; advise about possible scarring
  - Dichloroacetic acid applied sparingly; advise about burning sensation after application

CAVEATS AND PITFALLS
- Removal for cosmetic reasons only.

ACRODERMATITIS ENTEROPATHICA

ALTERNATE DISEASE NAME
- Zinc deficiency syndrome
- Zinc depletion syndrome
- Transient symptomatic zinc deficiency
- Self-limiting acrodermatitis enteropathica
- Danbolt-Closs syndrome

HISTORY
- Symptoms occur within the first few months after birth, often shortly after discontinuation of breast-feeding
- Development of marked irritability, variable diarrhea & nonspecific dermatitis

PHYSICAL EXAMINATION
- Presents as red patches and/or scaly plaques
- Evolution into crusted, vesiculobullous, erosive & pustular plaques
- Periorificial & acral distribution on face, scalp, hands, feet & anogenital areas
- Alopecia of scalp & eyebrows

DIFFERENTIAL DIAGNOSIS
- Seborrheic dermatitis
- Atopic dermatitis
- Biotin & multiple decarboxylase deficiencies
- Essential fatty acid deficiencies
- Langerhans cell histiocytosis
- Mucocutaneous candidiasis
- Glucagonoma syndrome
- Cystic fibrosis

LABORATORY WORK-UP
- Plasma or serum zinc level

MANAGEMENT
- Zinc supplementation

SPECIFIC THERAPY
- Elemental zinc 50 mg PO per day

CAVEATS AND PITFALLS
- May develop secondary bacterial or candidal skin infection.
- Lifetime zinc therapy needed.

ACROKERATOELASTOIDOSIS

ALTERNATE DISEASE NAME
- Acrokeratoelastoidosis marginalis

- Acrokeratoelastoidosis of Costa
- Acrokeratoderma hereditarium punctatum
- Hereditary papulotranslucent acrokeratoderma

HISTORY
- Gradual onset of small papules over margins of hands & feet, usually after puberty
- Remains stable once fully developed

PHYSICAL EXAMINATION
- Keratotic translucent papules that arise on margins of hands & feet, in a linear distribution

DIFFERENTIAL DIAGNOSIS
- Keratoelastoidosis marginalis
- Focal acral hyperkeratosis
- Flat warts
- Acrokeratosis verruciformis of Hopf

LABORATORY WORK-UP
- None

MANAGEMENT
- No effective therapy

SPECIFIC THERAPY
- None

CAVEATS AND PITFALLS
- None

ACROPUSTULOSIS OF INFANCY

ALTERNATE DISEASE NAME
- Infantile acropustulosis

HISTORY
- Occurs most often in black infants
- Onset between birth & 2 years
- Individual episodes last 7–15 days & recur at 2- to 4-week intervals
- Spontaneous permanent remission by 2–3 years of age

PHYSICAL EXAMINATION
- Recurrent crops of small vesicles that evolve into pustules
- Lesions on palms, soles & dorsal aspects of distal extremities

DIFFERENTIAL DIAGNOSIS
- Erythema toxicum neonatorum
- Transient neonatal pustular melanosis
- Dyshidrosis
- Scabies
- Pyoderma
- Subcorneal pustular dermatosis
- Pustular psoriasis
- Cutaneous candidiasis
- Fire ant bites
- Hand-foot-and-mouth disease

LABORATORY WORK-UP
- Bacterial culture of pustule to rule out pyoderma

MANAGEMENT
- Topical corticosteroids
- Dapsone in severe cases

SPECIFIC THERAPY
- Fluocinonide 0.05% cream applied BID
- Dapsone 1–2 mg/kg PO daily

CAVEATS AND PITFALLS
- Check CBC Q2–3 weeks for 10–12 weeks w/ dapsone to detect rare pancytopenia.
- Check G6PD level before starting therapy.

ACTINIC KERATOSIS

ALTERNATE DISEASE NAME
- Solar keratosis
- Senile keratosis

HISTORY
- Develops on sun-exposed skin of fair-skinned pts w/ significant sun exposure

- May flare during periods of depressed immunity
- Identifies person at risk for subsequent squamous cell carcinoma of skin

PHYSICAL EXAMINATION
- Poorly defined, red, scaly, nonsubstantive papule on sun-exposed areas of skin
- Occurs in the milieu of sun-damaged skin (wrinkling, dyspigmentation)

DIFFERENTIAL DIAGNOSIS
- Squamous cell carcinoma
- Bowen's disease
- Seborrheic keratosis
- Wart
- Lichenoid keratosis
- Cutaneous lupus erythematosus
- Lentigo maligna

LABORATORY WORK-UP
- Biopsy to rule out squamous cell carcinoma in questionable cases

MANAGEMENT
- Destructive modalities
- Fluorouracil cream for multiple lesions
- Photodynamic therapy for multiple lesions
- Imiquimod cream for multiple lesions

SPECIFIC THERAPY
- Destruction by liquid nitrogen cryotherapy; advise about post-inflammatory hypopigmentation
- Destruction by electrodesiccation & curettage
- Destruction by chemical peel
- Fluorouracil 0.5–5% cream applied QD-BID for 30 days; advise about irritation
- Photodynamic therapy using aminolevulinic acid & blue light
- Imiquimod 5% cream BIW for up to 16 wks

CAVEATS AND PITFALLS
- Recurrence common after liquid nitrogen cryotherapy.

- Advise about extreme irritation w/ fluorouracil cream & imiquimod cream.
- Extreme pain possible w/ photodynamic therapy.

ACUTE FEBRILE NEUTROPHILIC DERMATOSIS

ALTERNATE DISEASE NAME
- Sweet syndrome
- Neutrophilic dermatitis

HISTORY
- Often preceded by upper respiratory or GI infection
- Each crop of lesions often preceded by fever, myalgias, arthralgias & headache
- May be associated w/ underlying systemic inflammatory disorder or leukemia

PHYSICAL EXAMINATION
- Erythematous or violaceous papules or nodules, which may coalesce into circinate or arcuate plaques or may be studded w/ pustules
- Lesions may appear almost vesicular because of subepidermal edema

DIFFERENTIAL DIAGNOSIS
- Vasculitis
- Erythema multiforme
- Pyoderma gangrenosum
- Leukemia cutis
- Behçet disease
- Bowel-associated dermatitis-arthritis syndrome
- Neutrophilic rheumatoid dermatitis
- Cutaneous metastasis
- Acute hemorrhagic edema of childhood

LABORATORY WORK-UP
- Complete blood count w/ differential
- Bone marrow aspiration is indicated if CBC findings are abnormal
- Skin biopsy for light microscopic exam

MANAGEMENT
- Systemic corticosteroids
- Corticosteroid-sparing agents
- Intralesional corticosteroids for local control

SPECIFIC THERAPY
- Prednisone 1 mg/kg PO daily
- Corticosteroid-sparing agents
  - Dapsone 100–200 mg PO daily
  - Cyclosporine 3–5 mg/kg PO daily
- Triamcinolone 3–5 mg/kg intralesional

CAVEATS AND PITFALLS
- Order baseline chest radiograph, TB skin test, bone mineral density if chronic corticosteroids are considered.

ALOPECIA AREATA

ALTERNATE DISEASE NAME
- Autoimmune alopecia

HISTORY
- Abrupt localized, patterned hair loss
- May occur in pts w/ family history of autoimmune phenomena

PHYSICAL EXAMINATION
- Non-scarring, non-inflammatory, patterned alopecia
- One or many round to oval bald patches
- Exclamation point hairs (i.e., hairs tapered near proximal end)
- Most common in the scalp, but possible in any hair-bearing area

DIFFERENTIAL DIAGNOSIS
- Androgenetic alopecia
- Telogen effluvium
- Tinea capitis
- Telogen effluvium
- Trichotillomania
- Pseudopelade of Brocq
- Lichen planopilaris
- Syphilis

LABORATORY WORK-UP
- None, in the absence of systemic signs & symptoms of autoimmune diseases

MANAGEMENT
- Topical, intralesional or systemic corticosteroids
- Topical sensitizing agents or irritants
- Photochemotherapy
- Systemic immune modulators

SPECIFIC THERAPY
- Localized disease
  - Triamcinolone 2–4 mg/mL intralesional
  - High-potency topical corticosteroids such as clobetasol 0.05% cream applied BID
- Widespread disease
  - Prednisone, 0.5–1 mg/kg per day PO
  - Anthralin 0.5–1% cream applied daily
  - Topical immunotherapy w/ squaric acid
  - Photochemotherapy
  - Cyclosporine 3–5 mg/kg PO daily

CAVEATS AND PITFALLS
- Hair may fall out again after tapering prednisone.
- Squaric acid will produce skin irritation.
- Anthralin will stain the skin.

AMALGAM TATTOO

ALTERNATE DISEASE NAME
- None

HISTORY
- Asymptomatic oral lesions, often first noted after dental exam
- Occurs after amalgam dental fillings placed

PHYSICAL EXAMINATION
- Painless, blue/gray/black macule without surrounding erythema
- Most frequently found on gingival or alveolar mucosa

DIFFERENTIAL DIAGNOSIS
- Mucosal melanosis
- Nevus
- Melanoma
- Venous lake
- Medication reaction
- Hemangioma
- Peutz-Jeghers syndrome

LABORATORY WORK-UP
- Skin biopsy, only if melanoma is a consideration

MANAGEMENT
- No therapy indicated

SPECIFIC THERAPY
- None

CAVEATS AND PITFALLS
- None

ANAGEN EFFLUVIUM

ALTERNATE DISEASE NAME
- Chemotherapy-induced alopecia

HISTORY
- Begins 7–14 days after chemotherapy pulse or after exposure to toxic chemical
- Most prominent w/ doxorubicin, cyclophosphamide & the nitrosoureas

PHYSICAL EXAMINATION
- Diffuse, non-inflammatory, non-scarring alopecia
- Most notable over scalp & beard area

DIFFERENTIAL DIAGNOSIS
- Telogen effluvium
- Androgenetic alopecia
- Malnutrition
- Traction alopecia

- Follicular degeneration syndrome
- Alopecia mucinosa
- Alopecia secondary to thyroid disease

LABORATORY WORK-UP
- None

MANAGEMENT
- No therapy indicated for this self-limited problem

SPECIFIC THERAPY
- None

CAVEATS AND PITFALLS
- None

ANDROGENETIC ALOPECIA

ALTERNATE DISEASE NAME
- Common baldness
- Familial baldness
- Hereditary baldness

HISTORY
- Gradual onset of asymptomatic hair thinning in the temporal area in men & diffusely in women
- Genetic component in both men & women

PHYSICAL EXAMINATION
- Progressive, patterned, non-inflammatory, non-scarring alopecia of the scalp

DIFFERENTIAL DIAGNOSIS
- Telogen effluvium
- Alopecia areata
- Virilizing disorders in women
- Anagen effluvium
- Thyroid disease
- Iron deficiency

LABORATORY WORK-UP
- Scalp biopsy only if there is a question about the diagnosis

- Work-up for systemic illness associated w/ alopecia only if there are other signs & symptoms of disease
- Androgen profile only if virilization is suspected
  - Serum free testosterone
  - Sex hormone binding globulin
  - Luteinizing hormone
  - Follicle-stimulating hormone

MANAGEMENT
- Hair loss prevention
- New hair growth treatments

SPECIFIC THERAPY
- Minoxidil 5% solution applied twice daily. Advise about 6-month trial needed to assess response
- Finasteride 1 mg PO daily (men only). Advise that this may stabilize hair loss without causing increased hair growth.
- Spironolactone 100 mg PO twice daily (women only)
- Hair transplantation

CAVEATS AND PITFALLS
- Only 15–20% of people get meaningful hair growth w/ minoxidil.
- Finasteride better at maintaining hair than regrowing it.

ANGIOFIBROMA

ALTERNATE DISEASE NAME
- Fibrous papule of nose & face
- Pearly penile papule
- Oral fibroma
- Adenoma sebaceum

HISTORY
- Gradual onset of asymptomatic skin lesion(s)

PHYSICAL EXAMINATION
- Solitary or multiple firm, discrete, flesh-colored-to-telangiectatic papules

DIFFERENTIAL DIAGNOSIS
- Melanocytic nevus
- Basal cell carcinoma

- Benign cutaneous appendage tumors
- Acne vulgaris
- Rosacea
- Flat warts
- Molluscum contagiosum
- Folliculitis
- Cherry angioma
- Sarcoidosis
- Granuloma annulare

LABORATORY WORK-UP
- Skin biopsy only if diagnosis is in doubt

MANAGEMENT
- Surgical removal

SPECIFIC THERAPY
- Shave removal
- Destruction by electrodesiccation & curettage
- CO_2 laser vaporization
- Dermabrasion

CAVEATS AND PITFALLS
- None

ANGIOKERATOMA OF THE SCROTUM (VULVA)

ALTERNATE DISEASE NAME
- Angiokeratoma of Fordyce
- Fordyce angiokeratoma
- Angiokeratoma scroti
- Angiokeratoma of the vulva
- Angiokeratoma vulvae

HISTORY
- Adult onset
- Asymptomatic

PHYSICAL EXAMINATION
- Solitary or multiple friable 2- to 3-mm red to blue papules on scrotum or labia majora

DIFFERENTIAL DIAGNOSIS
- Angiokeratoma corporis diffusum
- Pyogenic granuloma
- Cherry angioma
- Lymphangioma
- Seborrheic keratosis
- Wart
- Blue rubber bleb nevus

LABORATORY WORK-UP
- Skin biopsy only if diagnosis is in doubt

MANAGEMENT
- Surgical destruction for cosmetic purposes only

SPECIFIC THERAPY
- Destruction by electrodesiccation & curettage
- Laser therapy w/ copper vapor or pulsedye laser

CAVEATS AND PITFALLS
- New lesions may arise after older ones have been destroyed.

ANGIOKERATOSIS CORPORIS DIFFUSUM

ALTERNATE DISEASE NAME
- Fabry disease
- Fabry-Anderson disease
- Fabry syndrome

HISTORY
- Pain & paresthesias of extremities noted in first decade
- Gradual onset of asymptomatic skin lesions
- Progressive renal insufficiency
- Coronary artery disease & cerebrovascular disease

PHYSICAL EXAMINATION
- Multiple red to violaceous papules w/ a predilection for scrotum, penis, lower back, thighs, hips, buttocks & lips
- Lesions may become slightly verrucous over time
- Lesions typically spare face, scalp & ears

- Hypohidrosis
- Lenticular opacities

DIFFERENTIAL DIAGNOSIS
- Angiokeratoma of the scrotum
- Adult-type beta-galactosidase deficiency
- Aspartylglucosaminuria
- Adult-onset variant of alpha-N-acetylgalactosaminidase deficiency
- Fucosidosis
- Sialidosis

LABORATORY WORK-UP
- Plasma or leukocyte alpha-galactosidase level
- Urine polarizing microscopy, evaluating for birefringent lipid globules ("Maltese crosses")
- Urine oligosaccharide assays to rule out other lysosomal storage diseases
- Skin biopsy of suspect angiokeratoma

MANAGEMENT
- No specific therapy for underlying genetic defect
- Destructive modalities for individual skin lesions

SPECIFIC THERAPY
- Destruction of individual lesions w/ electrodesiccation & curettage
- Laser therapy w/ copper vapor or pulse dye laser

CAVEATS AND PITFALLS
- None

ANGIOLYMPHOID HYPERPLASIA WITH EOSINOPHILIA

ALTERNATE DISEASE NAME
- Epithelioid hemangioma
- Histiocytoid hemangioma
- Pseudopyogenic granuloma
- Papular angioplasia
- Inflammatory angiomatous nodule

HISTORY
- Onset in middle age
- More common in women
- Occasionally associated w/ minor trauma

PHYSICAL EXAMINATION
- Enlarging, dome-shaped, red to brown, solitary or multiple papules or nodules, usually in head & neck area
- May be associated w/ pain or pruritus
- Peripheral eosinophilia in 20% of cases

DIFFERENTIAL DIAGNOSIS
- Pyogenic granuloma
- Hemangioma
- Granuloma faciale
- Insect bite reaction
- Melanoma
- Pseudolymphoma
- Lymphoma
- Kaposi's sarcoma

LABORATORY WORK-UP
- Skin biopsy
- Eosinophil count

MANAGEMENT
- Surgical excision
- Superficial orthovoltage radiation
- Intralesional corticosteroids
- Liquid nitrogen cryotherapy

SPECIFIC THERAPY
- Elliptical excision
- Triamcinolone 3–5 mg/mL intralesional; repeat in 6 wks as needed

CAVEATS AND PITFALLS
- None

ANHIDROTIC ECTODERMAL DYSPLASIA

ALTERNATE DISEASE NAME
- Hypohidrotic ectodermal dysplasia
- Christ-Siemens-Touraine syndrome

HISTORY
- Marked heat intolerance from birth
- Minimal sweating

PHYSICAL EXAMINATION
- Newborns may have collodion membrane or marked scaling
- Pyrexia secondary to inadequate sweating
- Abnormal facies
- Sparse hair & abnormal nails
- Skin dryness
- Markedly dystrophic teeth w/ early caries

DIFFERENTIAL DIAGNOSIS
- Hidrotic ectodermal dysplasia
- Congenital ichthyosis
- Rapp-Hodgkin syndrome
- Rosselli-Giulienetti syndrome
- Ectrodactyly ectodermal dysplasia clefting syndrome

LABORATORY WORK-UP
- Sweat testing w/ starch iodine, only in carefully controlled environment

MANAGEMENT
- Control ambient temperature
- Regular dental care

SPECIFIC THERAPY
- Emollients for dry skin, applied at least BID

CAVEATS AND PITFALLS
- Pts are very susceptible to hyperthermia.

ANTHRAX, CUTANEOUS

ALTERNATE DISEASE NAME
- Malignant pustule
- Wool sorter's disease
- Black bane
- Charbon
- Murrain
- Black blood

HISTORY
- Transmitted to humans by direct contact w/ infected materials or from contaminated fomites (clothing, etc.)
- Incubation period is 1–7 days (usually 2–5) after skin exposure.

PHYSICAL EXAMINATION
- Primarily affects exposed skin surfaces
- Starts as pruritic papule that enlarges in 24–48 hours to form an ulcer
- Evolves into a black eschar; which lasts for 7–14 days before separating & leaving a permanent scar
- Regional lymphadenopathy, which may be present for weeks after the ulceration heals

DIFFERENTIAL DIAGNOSIS
- Staphylococcal pyoderma
- Atypical mycobacterial infection
- Sporotrichosis
- Bubonic plague
- Leishmaniasis
- Tularemia
- Syphilis
- North American blastomycosis
- Cat-scratch disease
- Cowpox
- Orf
- Milker's nodule

LABORATORY WORK-UP
- Gram stain & culture and/or antibody test of vesicle fluid
- Skin biopsy

MANAGEMENT
- Systemic antibiotics
- Vaccine prophylaxis for those at risk for infection

SPECIFIC THERAPY
- Penicillin 250–500 mg PO for up to 60 days in event of bioterrorism
- Doxycycline 100 mg PO BID for up to 60 days in event of bioterrorism

CAVEATS AND PITFALLS
- Contact public health authorities if this diagnosis is suspected.

ANTIPHOSPHOLIPID SYNDROME

ALTERNATE DISEASE NAME
- Antiphospholipid antibody syndrome
- Anticardiolipin syndrome
- Anticardiolipin antibody syndrome

HISTORY
- Recurrent fetal loss
- Recurrent thrombotic events, including CVA, pulmonary embolism & thrombophlebitis, often at early age
- May be associated w/ lupus erythematosus

PHYSICAL EXAMINATION
- Livedo reticularis
- Superficial thrombophlebitis
- Leg ulcers
- Painful purpura
- Splinter hemorrhages in nail beds
- Raynaud's phenomenon

DIFFERENTIAL DIAGNOSIS
- Systemic necrotizing vasculitis
- Hypercoagulable state from other causes such as malignancy
- Endocarditis
- Disseminated intravascular coagulation

- Thrombotic thrombocytopenic purpura
- Atherosclerotic vascular disease
- Cholesterol emboli

LABORATORY WORK-UP
- Coagulation profile
- Rheumatic disease serologies
- Anticardiolipin antibodies & lupus anticoagulant
- Complete blood count

MANAGEMENT
- Eliminate thrombosis risk factors such as oral contraceptives, smoking, hypertension & hyperlipidemia
- Long-term anticoagulation

SPECIFIC THERAPY
- Aspirin 81 mg PO per day, especially in women w/ recurrent fetal loss
- Warfarin: 2–15 mg PO per day
- Enoxaparin: 1 mg/kg subcutaneously twice daily

CAVEATS AND PITFALLS
- Suspect this condition in those w/ multiple spontaneous abortions or unexplained recurrent deep vein thrombophlebitis.

APHTHOUS STOMATITIS

ALTERNATE DISEASE NAME
- Aphthae
- Recurrent aphthous stomatitis
- Recurrent aphthous ulcers
- Canker sores
- Periadenitis mucosa necrotica recurrens

HISTORY
- Recurrent episodes of painful ulcerations in the mouth
- Episodes may be related to psychological stress, systemic illness, local trauma to oral cavity

PHYSICAL EXAMINATION
- Aphthae minor
  - Recurrent, discrete, painful, punched-out ulcers, which occur on the labial & buccal mucosa & the floor of the mouth
  - Lesions heal without scarring in 7–10 days
- Aphthae major
  - Large oval ulcers
  - Multiple lesions, often presenting simultaneously
  - Healing after 4–8 wks

DIFFERENTIAL DIAGNOSIS
- Herpes simplex virus infection
- Erythema multiforme
- Lichen planus
- Pemphigus vulgaris
- Traumatic ulceration
- Behçet's syndrome
- Oral cancer
- Hand-foot-and-mouth disease
- Contact dermatitis
- Lupus erythematosus
- Paraneoplastic pemphigus
- Reiter syndrome
- Syphilis
- Cyclic neutropenia

LABORATORY WORK-UP
- Culture of ulcer to rule out herpes simplex virus infection
- Biopsy to rule out pemphigus vulgaris or oral cancer

MANAGEMENT
- Topical soothing or anesthetic agents
- Systemic corticosteroids
- Immune modulators

SPECIFIC THERAPY
- Topical therapy
  - Kaopectate applied to ulcer 3 or 4 times per day
  - Zilactin gel applied 4 or 5 times per day

- ➤ High-potency topical corticosteroids, such as fluocinonide 0.05% gel applied TID
- ➤ Viscous lidocaine applied as needed
- ➤ Amlexanox 5% paste applied 4 times daily
- ➤ Tetracycline suspension (250-mg capsule contents suspended in 5 mL water) applied to ulcers 4 times daily
- ■ Systemic therapy (mostly for aphthae major)
  - ➤ Thalidomide 100–300 mg PO per day
  - ➤ Prednisone 1 mg/kg PO per day
  - ➤ Colchicine 0.6–1.8 mg PO per day
  - ➤ Azathioprine 2–3 mg/kg PO per day

CAVEATS AND PITFALLS
- ■ Advise about possible peripheral neuropathy w/ thalidomide.
- ■ Use prednisone for no longer than 21 days per course of therapy.

APLASIA CUTIS CONGENITA

ALTERNATE DISEASE NAME
- ■ Congenital ulcer of the newborn
- ■ Congenital localized absence of skin
- ■ Streeter's spots

HISTORY
- ■ Lesion(s) present at birth, usually on the scalp
- ■ May be associated w/ other congenital anomalies

PHYSICAL EXAMINATION
- ■ Stellate, linear or oval, sharply demarcated ulceration, atrophic scar or bulla, most often over posterior scalp
- ■ Multiple lesions may occur over extremities, trunk, buttocks
- ■ Spontaneous healing in 1–3 months, but slower healing w/ underlying bony defects

DIFFERENTIAL DIAGNOSIS
- ■ Traumatic injury from scalp electrode, etc.
- ■ Congenital varicella
- ■ Focal dermal hypoplasia
- ■ Epidermolysis bullosa
- ■ Volkmann's ischemic contracture

LABORATORY WORK-UP
■ None

MANAGEMENT
■ Surgery only for large, non-healing defects

SPECIFIC THERAPY
■ Surgical reconstruction w/ skin grafting or advancement flaps
  for closure

CAVEATS AND PITFALLS
■ Avoid surgical correction unless the defect does not heal over
  many months.

ARGYRIA

ALTERNATE DISEASE NAME
■ Argyrosis

HISTORY
■ Exposure to silver-containing compounds from occupation,
  ingestion of alternative medicinal therapies
■ Chronic topical silver sulfadiazine therapy on extensive burns or
  other wounds

PHYSICAL EXAMINATION
■ Diffuse, slate-gray pigmentation of gingiva & oral mucosa
■ Sun-exposed skin, sclera & nails may be more intensely involved

DIFFERENTIAL DIAGNOSIS
■ Hyperpigmentation from other drugs, such as minocycline, gold
  or phenothiazine derivative
■ Cyanosis
■ Diffuse melanosis from metastatic melanoma

LABORATORY WORK-UP
■ Skin biopsy, looking for silver granules

MANAGEMENT
■ Discontinue exposure to silver
■ Sun avoidance
■ Chelating agents

SPECIFIC THERAPY
- Dimercaprol (BAL) only w/ severe toxicity

CAVEATS AND PITFALLS
- Question pt about use of silver as alternative form of therapy for various ailments.
- May be purchased over the Internet.

ARSENICAL KERATOSIS

ALTERNATE DISEASE NAME
- None

HISTORY
- Chronic arsenic exposure through contaminated drinking water or occupational exposure

PHYSICAL EXAMINATION
- Punctate, non-tender, hard, yellowish, often symmetric, corn-like papules
- Occurs mainly on palms & soles & over pressure points
- Lesions may coalesce to form large, verrucous plaques

DIFFERENTIAL DIAGNOSIS
- Keratosis palmaris et plantaris
- Clavus (corn)
- Wart
- Psoriasis of palms & soles
- Pityriasis rubra pilaris
- Nevoid basal cell carcinoma syndrome
- Porokeratosis
- Lichen planus
- Darier's disease
- Bazex syndrome

LABORATORY WORK-UP
- None

MANAGEMENT
- Chelation therapy for severe toxicity
- Retinoids
- Destructive modalities for individual lesions

SPECIFIC THERAPY
- Acitretin 25–50 mg PO per day indefinitely
- Destructive therapies
  - Electrosurgery
  - Liquid nitrogen cryotherapy
  - Laser vaporization

CAVEATS AND PITFALLS
- Keratoses may be precursor to squamous cell carcinoma.

ASHY DERMATOSIS

ALTERNATE DISEASE NAME
- Erythema dyschromicum perstans
- Ashy dermatosis of Ramirez
- Lichen pigmentosus
- Dermatosis cenicienta
- Erythema chronicum figuratum melanodermicum

HISTORY
- Slow development of asymptomatic gray lesions
- Usually no pre-existing dermatosis

PHYSICAL EXAMINATION
- Asymptomatic, gray-blue patches of variable shape & size, distributed symmetrically on face, trunk, upper extremities
- Elevated red border in early stages
- Oral cavity & genitalia spared

DIFFERENTIAL DIAGNOSIS
- Lichen planus
- Lichenoid drug eruption
- Leprosy
- Hemochromatosis
- Pinta

LABORATORY WORK-UP
- Skin biopsy to confirm diagnosis

MANAGEMENT
- No universally effective therapy
- Spontaneous remissions without treatment

SPECIFIC THERAPY
- Clofazimine 100 mg PO every other day if <40 kg in weight; clofazimine 100 mg every day if >40 kg in weight
- Dapsone 100 mg PO per day for 3 months

CAVEATS AND PITFALLS
- Treatments of very limited utility.

ATOPIC DERMATITIS

ALTERNATE DISEASE NAME
- Atopic eczema
- Infantile eczema
- Besnier's prurigo

HISTORY
- Onset before age 5 years in 90% of cases
- Concomitant asthma & respiratory allergies
- Common family history of atopy

PHYSICAL EXAMINATION
- Marked pruritus, often starting in first few months of life
- Dry skin
- Lichenified plaques w/ epithelial disruption
  - ➤ Occurs on face in infancy
  - ➤ Presents in flexural creases, trunk, diaper area by 1 year of age
  - ➤ Occurs over distal extremities later in life
- Scalp scale & erythema, usually after 3 months of age

DIFFERENTIAL DIAGNOSIS
- Seborrheic dermatitis
- Contact dermatitis
- Stasis dermatitis
- Nummular eczema
- Scabies
- Mycosis fungoides
- Dermatophytosis

LABORATORY WORK-UP
- None

MANAGEMENT
- Topical corticosteroids
- Emollients
- Topical macrolide immunomodulators
- Systemic corticosteroids
- Nonsteroidal immunosuppressives
  - ➤ Used only in severe, recalcitrant disease
- Phototherapy

SPECIFIC THERAPY
- Mid-potency topical corticosteroids, such as triamcinolone 0.1% cream or ointment applied BID
- Prednisone 1 mg/kg PO QD for no longer than 21 days
  - ➤ Caution: use only w/ extreme flares
- Topical macrolide immunomodulators
  - ➤ Tacrolimus 0.3% or 1% ointment applied BID
  - ➤ Pimecrolimus 1% cream applied BID
- Systemic immunosuppressives
  - ➤ Azathioprine 2–3 mg/kg PO QD
  - ➤ Cyclosporine 3–5 mg/kg PO QD
  - ➤ Methotrexate 5–10 mg PO q 7 days
- Antihistamines, such as diphenhydramine 25–50 mg PO QHS for nighttime sedation
- UVB phototherapy
- Emollients applied at least twice daily, particularly in winter

CAVEATS AND PITFALLS
- Topical immunomodulators are equivalent in potency to mid-potency topical corticosteroids & are mainly useful for facial lesions.
- Prednisone should be used for no more than 3 wks per course.
- Consider systemic immunosuppressives in adults instead of long-term systemic corticosteroids.

ATYPICAL FIBROXANTHOMA

ALTERNATE DISEASE NAME
- Superficial variant of malignant fibrous histiocytoma
- Paradoxical fibrosarcoma

- Pseudosarcoma
- Pseudosarcomatous reticulohistiocytoma
- Pseudosarcomatous dermatofibroma

HISTORY
- Usually occurs in elderly people
- Presents as rapidly growing nodule on sun-exposed skin

PHYSICAL EXAMINATION
- Firm, solitary, eroded or ulcerated papule or nodule
- Occurs most often on ear, nose, cheek

DIFFERENTIAL DIAGNOSIS
- Squamous cell carcinoma
- Basal cell carcinoma
- Pyogenic granuloma
- Melanoma
- Merkel cell carcinoma
- Cutaneous metastasis
- Leiomyosarcoma
- Dermatofibrosarcoma protuberans

LABORATORY WORK-UP
- Diagnostic skin biopsy

MANAGEMENT
- Surgical excision

SPECIFIC THERAPY
- Mohs micrographic surgery
- Elliptical excision

CAVEATS AND PITFALLS
- Tumor has low metastatic potential.
- Incomplete excision often results in local recurrence.

ATYPICAL MOLE

ALTERNATE DISEASE NAME
- Dysplastic nevus

- Clark's nevus
- Dysplastic mole
- Atypical melanocytic nevus
- Active junctional nevus
- B-K mole

HISTORY
- Present in 5% of otherwise healthy Caucasians
- Familial predisposition in some cases
- Melanoma more common if there is familial melanoma history

PHYSICAL EXAMINATION
- Variable features w/ some or all of the following:
  - Asymmetrical conformation
  - Irregular border, which can fade into surrounding skin
  - Variable coloration, w/ shades of tan, brown, black, red
  - Diameter >6 mm
  - Elevated center; feathered, flat border

DIFFERENTIAL DIAGNOSIS
- Melanoma
- Compound nevus
- Seborrheic keratosis
- Dermatofibroma
- Wart

LABORATORY WORK-UP
- Diagnostic biopsy if melanoma is suspected

MANAGEMENT
- No therapy indicated
- Periodic follow-up to evaluate for possible melanoma development, particularly in familial cases

SPECIFIC THERAPY
- None

CAVEATS AND PITFALLS
- Increased melanoma potential if there is family history of melanoma & personal history of atypical moles.
- Little reason to remove all atypical moles prophylactically.

BACILLARY ANGIOMATOSIS

ALTERNATE DISEASE NAME
- Disseminated cat-scratch disease
- Epithelioid angiomatosis
- Bartonellosis
- Bacillary ailuronosis

HISTORY
- Caused by infection w/ *Bartonella species*, *B henselae* & *B quintana*
- Occurs after exposure to flea-infested cats or human body louse
- Occurs mainly in HIV-infected individuals

PHYSICAL EXAMINATION
- Globular cherry-red papules or nodules
- Violaceous nodules & plaques
- Subcutaneous papules or nodules, w/ or w/out ulceration

DIFFERENTIAL DIAGNOSIS
- Kaposi's sarcoma
- Pyogenic granuloma
- Hemangioma
- Angiokeratoma
- Glomangioma
- Gram-positive bacterial abscess
- Melanoma

LABORATORY WORK-UP
- Skin biopsy w/ Warthin-Starry tissue staining
- Culture of skin biopsy material

MANAGEMENT
- Systemic antibiotics

SPECIFIC THERAPY
- Erythromycin 500 mg PO 4 times per day for 3 wks
- Azithromycin 500 mg PO on day 1, 250 mg PO on days 2–5
- Clarithromycin 250 mg PO twice per day for 3 wks
- Doxycycline 100 mg PO twice per day for 3 wks

CAVEATS AND PITFALLS
- House cats are vectors of disease.

BASAL CELL CARCINOMA

ALTERNATE DISEASE NAME
- Basal cell epithelioma
- Basalioma

HISTORY
- Slow-growing lesion, often in sun-exposed skin
- Bleeding after minor trauma

PHYSICAL EXAMINATION
- Nodular variant
  - Pearly, translucent papule w/ central depression, erosion or ulceration
  - Rolled borders
  - Surface telangiectasia
- Pigmented variant
  - Small spots of gray or blue pigment in addition to features described for nodular variant
- Morpheaform variant
  - Poorly demarcated, sclerotic plaque or papule
- Superficial variant
  - Pink to brown, scaly plaque or papule
  - May have annular configuration

DIFFERENTIAL DIAGNOSIS
- Squamous cell carcinoma
- Sebaceous gland hyperplasia
- Fibrous papule
- Melanocytic nevus
- Wart
- Appendage tumor
- Seborrheic keratosis
- Carcinoma in situ

LABORATORY WORK-UP
- Diagnostic skin biopsy

MANAGEMENT
- Destructive modalities
- Radiation therapy
- Surgical excision

SPECIFIC THERAPY

- Primary tumor in anatomically insensitive sites
  - ➤ Destruction by electrodesiccation & curettage
  - ➤ Cryotherapy
- Elliptical excision
- Orthovoltage radiation therapy
- Recurrent tumor or tumors in anatomically sensitive sites
  - ➤ Mohs micrographic surgery

CAVEATS AND PITFALLS

- Repeat treatment w/ destructive modality after recurrence; commonly recurs again.

BASAL CELL NEVUS SYNDROME

ALTERNATE DISEASE NAME

- Nevoid basal cell carcinoma syndrome
- Gorlin syndrome
- Gorlin-Goltz syndrome
- Bifid-rib basal-cell nevus syndrome

HISTORY

- Family history of similar signs & symptoms
- Multiple basal cell carcinomas, often early in life
- History of one or more skeletal anomalies

PHYSICAL EXAMINATION

- Pitting of palms or soles
- Multiple basal cell carcinomas
- Jaw cysts
- Cleft palate
- Coarse facies w/ milia, frontal bossing, widened nasal bridge, mandibular prognathia
- Ocular findings include strabismus, dystrophic canthorum & ocular hypertelorism
- Calcification of falx cerebri
- Orthopedic anomalies include spine & rib abnormalities, high-arched eyebrows & palate
- Kidney anomalies
- Hypogonadism in males

DIFFERENTIAL DIAGNOSIS
- Non-syndromic basal cell carcinoma
- Bazex syndrome
- Linear unilateral basal cell nevus w/ comedos
- Rasmussen syndrome

LABORATORY WORK-UP
- Skin biopsy of suspicious lesions
- Radiologic studies of suspected skeletal anomalies

MANAGEMENT
- Sun avoidance
- Surgical therapy of skin cancers
- Medical therapy for multiple skin malignancies

SPECIFIC THERAPY
- Surgical therapy
  - Primary tumor in anatomically insensitive sites
    - Destruction by electrodesiccation & curettage
    - Elliptical excision
    - Cryotherapy
  - Recurrent tumor or those in anatomically sensitive sites
    - Mohs micrographic surgery
- Medical therapy for multiple tumors
  - Fluorouracil 0.5–5% cream applied QD for at least 8 wks
  - Isotretinoin 1–2 mg/kg PO QD indefinitely

CAVEATS AND PITFALLS
- Avoid radiation therapy.
- Medical therapy may prevent new lesions but does little for established tumors.

BECKER'S NEVUS

ALTERNATE DISEASE NAME
- Becker melanosis
- Becker's pigmented hairy nevus
- Nevus spilus tardus
- Pigmented hairy epidermal nevus

HISTORY
- Onset in adolescence
- More common in males

PHYSICAL EXAMINATION
- Asymptomatic, irregular, tan to brown patch, most commonly located over chest, shoulder or back
- Coarse, brown to black hairs within & adjacent to patch
- May be associated w/ underlying smooth muscle hamartoma

DIFFERENTIAL DIAGNOSIS
- Melanoma
- Café-au-lait macule
- Congenital melanocytic nevus
- Nevus spilus
- Postinflammatory hyperpigmentation
- Albright's syndrome

LABORATORY WORK-UP
- Skin biopsy only if melanoma is diagnostic possibility

MANAGEMENT
- Surgical or laser therapy for cosmetic reasons only

SPECIFIC THERAPY
- Surgical excision
- Q-switched ruby laser ablation
- Q-switched neodymium: yttrium-aluminum-garnet (YAG) laser ablation

CAVEATS AND PITFALLS
- Incomplete clearing in most cases of laser ablation.

BEHÇET'S DISEASE

ALTERNATE DISEASE NAME
- Behçet's syndrome

HISTORY
- Most common in Middle East, Japan, Mediterranean basin
- Peak incidence in 3rd-4th decade
- Insidious onset of multisystem disorder

PHYSICAL EXAMINATION
- Mucocutaneous lesions
  - Recurrent oral & genital aphthae
  - Erythema nodosum
  - Subcutaneous thrombophlebitis
  - Folliculitis
  - Acne-like lesions
  - Cutaneous hypersensitivity (pathergy)
- Ocular lesions
  - Anterior or posterior uveitis
  - Chorioretinitis
- Arthritis without deformity or ankylosis
- GI lesions
  - Aphthae in esophagus & stomach
  - Ileocecal ulcers
  - Cramping abdominal pain
- Epididymitis
- CNS signs & symptoms

DIFFERENTIAL DIAGNOSIS
- Aphthous stomatitis
- Herpes simplex virus infection
- Acute febrile neutrophilic dermatosis
- Pemphigus vulgaris
- Lichen planus
- Inflammatory bowel disease
- Stevens-Johnson syndrome
- Lupus erythematosus

LABORATORY WORK-UP
- No absolutely diagnostic tests
  - Pathergy test: pustule arising at site of minor skin injury
  - Skin biopsy of pustule

MANAGEMENT
- Topical agents for aphthae
- Systemic immunomodulators & anti-inflammatory agents

SPECIFIC THERAPY
- Local therapy for aphthae

> Tetracycline suspension (250-mg capsule contents suspended in 5 mL water) applied to mouth or genital ulcers 4 times daily
> Fluocinonide 0.05% gel applied TID
> Kaopectate applied to ulcer 3 or 4 times per day
> Zilactin gel applied 4 or 5 times per day
> Viscous lidocaine applied as needed
> Amlexanox 5% paste applied 4 times daily
- Systemic therapy
  > Thalidomide 100–300 mg PO QD
  > Colchicine 0.6 mg PO 2 or 3 times per day
  > Prednisone 1 mg/kg PO QD
  > Azathioprine 2–3 mg/kg PO QD
  > Cyclosporine 3–5 mg/kg QD

CAVEATS AND PITFALLS
- Advise about possible peripheral neuropathy w/ thalidomide.
- If prednisone is to be used for >21 days per course of therapy, obtain baseline chest radiograph, TB skin test & bone mineral density determination.

BEJEL

ALTERNATE DISEASE NAME
- Non-venereal syphilis of children
- Endemic syphilis

HISTORY
- Endemic in rural parts of Africa & Middle East
- Transmitted by environmental factors
- Occurs mainly in small children

PHYSICAL EXAMINATION
- Primary stage
  > Painless ulcers within oral cavity
  > May appear as a nipple ulceration of a mother w/ a suckling infected child
- Secondary stage
  > Eroded plaques on lips, tongue, tonsils

- ➤ Angular stomatitis
- ➤ Vitamin B deficiency
- ➤ Condyloma lata-like lesions in anogenital area
- ➤ Generalized lymphadenopathy
- ➤ Painful osteoperiostitis in long bones
- ■ Tertiary (late) stage
  - ➤ Gummas that destroy bone & cartilage, particularly of the nose, producing saddle nose deformity

DIFFERENTIAL DIAGNOSIS
- ■ Syphilis
- ■ Yaws
- ■ Pinta
- ■ Leprosy
- ■ Cutaneous tuberculosis
- ■ Atopic dermatitis
- ■ Dermatophytosis
- ■ Psoriasis
- ■ Herpes simplex virus infection
- ■ Perlèche
- ■ Genital warts
- ■ Lupus erythematosus
- ■ Squamous cell carcinoma

LABORATORY WORK-UP
- ■ Darkfield examination of lesional fluid

MANAGEMENT
- ■ Systemic antibiotics

SPECIFIC THERAPY
- ■ Penicillin G benzathine 2.4 million units IM over age 10 yrs; 600,000 units as single IM injection under age 10 yrs
- ■ Tetracycline 500 mg PO QID for 15 days; not indicated under age 8 yrs
- ■ Erythromycin 500 mg PO QID for 15 days in adults; 8 mg/kg per day divided into 4 doses for 15 days in children

CAVEATS AND PITFALLS
- ■ None

BENIGN PIGMENTED PURPURA

ALTERNATE DISEASE NAME
- Pigmented purpuric dermatitis
- Pigmented purpuric eruption
- Subtypes
  - Schamberg disease (progressive pigmentary dermatosis)
  - Itching purpura of Loewenthal
  - Eczematid-like purpura of Doucas & Kapetanakis
  - Pigmented purpuric lichenoid dermatosis of Gougerot & Blum
  - Lichen aureus
  - Purpura annularis telangiectoides (Majocchi disease)

HISTORY
- Isolated finding in otherwise healthy people
- No known underlying cause

PHYSICAL EXAMINATION
- Reddish-brown, speckled discoloration in patches or plaques
- Schamberg variant
  - Cayenne pepper-like punctate petechial macules in a purpuric patch
- Lichen aureus variant
  - Golden-yellow patch
  - Most commonly on the leg
- Majocchi variant
  - Annular patches of purpura w/ telangiectasia
- Gougerot & Blum variant
  - Lichenoid surface change

DIFFERENTIAL DIAGNOSIS
- Thrombocytopenia
- Cryoglobulinemia or other vasculitis
- Cutaneous T-cell lymphoma
- Stasis-induced pigmentation
- Drug hypersensitivity reaction
- Scurvy

LABORATORY WORK-UP
- Platelet count to rule out thrombocytopenia
- Skin biopsy only if diagnosis of vasculitis is considered

MANAGEMENT
- Topical corticosteroids for symptomatic relief

SPECIFIC THERAPY
- Triamcinolone 0.1% cream applied BID

CAVEATS AND PITFALLS
- Common post-inflammatory hyperpigmentation

BERLOQUE DERMATITIS

ALTERNATE DISEASE NAME
- Berlock dermatitis
- Perfume phototoxicity
- Bergapten phototoxicity
- Bergamot phototoxicity

HISTORY
- Recent application of agent containing bergapten (5-MOP), such as colognes containing oil of bergamot

PHYSICAL EXAMINATION
- Erythema, edema, vesiculation, desquamation, pendant-like hyperpigmentation at sites of cologne application
- Often noted on lateral neck

DIFFERENTIAL DIAGNOSIS
- Contact dermatitis
- Postinflammatory hyperpigmentation
- Melasma
- Acanthosis nigricans
- Riehl melanosis

LABORATORY WORK-UP
- None

MANAGEMENT
- Sun avoidance to affected areas until pigmentation fades
- Discontinue use of offending agent

SPECIFIC THERAPY
- Avoidance of perfumes & colognes containing bergamot oil

CAVEATS AND PITFALLS
- Bergapten is a naturally occurring component of various fruits & plants, including figs, celery, lemon oil & Queen Anne's lace, all of which are capable of inducing bergapten photo-toxicity.

BLACK HEEL

ALTERNATE DISEASE NAME
- Calcaneal petechiae
- Talon noir
- Tennis heel
- Hyperkeratosis hemorrhagica
- Pseudochromhidrosis plantaris

HISTORY
- Occurs in those who participate in sports that involve frequent starts & stops, such as basketball, football, soccer, lacrosse, racquet sports

PHYSICAL EXAMINATION
- Multiple asymptomatic petechiae centrally aggregated w/ a few scattered satellite patches
- Located over posterior & posterolateral heel

DIFFERENTIAL DIAGNOSIS
- Melanoma
- Wart
- Nevus
- Lentigo

LABORATORY WORK-UP
- None

MANAGEMENT
- Protect heel from subsequent trauma

SPECIFIC THERAPY
- Pare lesion w/ a scalpel blade to remove heme pigment
- Protective heel pad or heel cup for prophylaxis

CAVEATS AND PITFALLS
- May be mistaken for melanoma; uniform speckled appearance differentiates these two entities.

BLISTERING DISTAL DACTYLITIS

ALTERNATE DISEASE NAME
- Blistering dactylitis

HISTORY
- Acute onset of tender lesions on fingers & toes
- Usually affects children
- Caused by group A streptococcal infection

PHYSICAL EXAMINATION
- Tender vesicle or bulla on an erythematous base
- Occurs over volar surface of affected digit
- No constitutional signs or symptoms

DIFFERENTIAL DIAGNOSIS
- Friction blister
- Herpetic whitlow
- Epidermolysis bullosa
- Burn or other trauma

LABORATORY WORK-UP
- Gram stain/culture of blister fluid

MANAGEMENT
- Surgical incision & drainage
- Systemic antibiotics

SPECIFIC THERAPY
- Penicillin G benzathine
  - 1.2 million units IM as single injection for adults
  - 0.3–0.6 million units IM for children <27 kg; 0.9 million units IM for children >27 kg

- Penicillin VK
  - ➤ 250–500 mg PO QID for 10 days in adults
  - ➤ 25–50 mg/kg PO QID for 10 days in children

CAVEATS AND PITFALLS
- None

BOTRYOMYCOSIS

ALTERNATE DISEASE NAME
- Granular bacteriosis
- Actinophytosis
- Bacterial pseudomycosis

HISTORY
- Associated w/ decreased immune status
- Most often caused by *S aureus*

PHYSICAL EXAMINATION
- Cutaneous or subcutaneous doughy nodules w/ ulcerations & draining sinuses
- Granular material extrudes from the lesions

DIFFERENTIAL DIAGNOSIS
- Mycetoma
- Actinomycosis
- Kerion
- Subcutaneous granuloma annulare
- Kaposi's sarcoma
- Lymphoma

LABORATORY WORK-UP
- KOH preparation, looking for coarse granules
- Gram stain/bacterial culture

MANAGEMENT
- Surgical debridement & excision
- Systemic antibiotics

SPECIFIC THERAPY
- Surgical therapy

- ➤ Debridement of necrotic material
- ➤ Elliptical excision
- ➤ CO_2 laser vaporization
- ■ Medical therapy
  - ➤ Dicloxacillin
    - 250–500 mg PO QID for 10 days in adults
    - 25–50 mg/kg PO 4 times per day for 7–10 days in children
  - ➤ Cephalexin
    - 250–500 mg PO QID for 10 days in adults
    - 25–100 mg/kg per day, divided into 4 doses, for 7–10 days in children

CAVEATS AND PITFALLS
- ■ Antibiotics alone are often insufficient w/ extensive necrotic material; requires surgical debridement.
- ■ 10–15% cross-reactivity between penicillin & cephalexin.

BOWEN'S DISEASE

ALTERNATE DISEASE NAME
- ■ Squamous cell carcinoma in situ
- ■ Bowen disease
- ■ Bowen's carcinoma

HISTORY
- ■ Slowly enlarging, asymptomatic lesion

PHYSICAL EXAMINATION
- ■ Red, scaly, non-substantive papule or plaque
- ■ Usually occurs on head & neck, but may appear on other sun-exposed areas, particularly the trunk

DIFFERENTIAL DIAGNOSIS
- ■ Actinic keratosis
- ■ Superficial basal cell carcinoma
- ■ Seborrheic keratosis
- ■ Tinea corporis
- ■ Lichenoid keratosis
- ■ Psoriasis
- ■ Lupus erythematosus
- ■ Extramammary Paget's disease

LABORATORY WORK-UP
- Skin biopsy

MANAGEMENT
- Destructive modalities
- Surgical excision
- Topical fluorouracil

SPECIFIC THERAPY
- Destruction by electrodesiccation & curettage
- Liquid nitrogen cryotherapy
- Elliptical excision
- Fluorouracil cream 0.5–5% applied 1 or 2 times daily for 6–8 wks

CAVEATS AND PITFALLS
- Common recurrences at margins; treat 2–5 mm beyond clinically obvious borders.

BOWENOID PAPULOSIS

ALTERNATE DISEASE NAME
- Viral keratosis
- Bowenoid papulosis of the penis
- Bowenoid papulosis of the genitalia

HISTORY
- Affects mainly sexually active adults
- Female sexual partners of men w/ this entity are at risk for cervical carcinoma

PHYSICAL EXAMINATION
- Solitary or multiple, pigmented papules w/ a flat to velvety surface
- Papules may coalesce into plaques
- Occurs most commonly on penile shaft in men or external genitalia in women

DIFFERENTIAL DIAGNOSIS
- Seborrheic keratosis
- Squamous cell carcinoma

- Melanocytic nevus
- Lichen planus

LABORATORY WORK-UP
- Skin biopsy to confirm clinical impression

MANAGEMENT
- Destructive modalities
- Topical anti-wart therapies

SPECIFIC THERAPY
- Destructive modalities
  - Electrodesiccation & curettage
  - Liquid nitrogen cryotherapy
  - CO_2 laser ablation
- Elliptical excision
- Medical therapy
  - Podofilox applied twice per day for 3 consecutive days per wk, up to 4 wks; advise about irritation
  - Fluorouracil 0.5–5% cream applied 1 or 2 times daily for 3–6 wks; advise about irritation

CAVEATS AND PITFALLS
- Safe sexual practices are critical to minimize chance of venereal spread of this carcinogenic virus.
- Sexual partners should be examined for possible cervical dysplasia.

BROMHIDROSIS

ALTERNATE DISEASE NAME
- Bromidrosis
- Apocrine bromhidrosis
- Osmidrosis

HISTORY
- Occurs after puberty
- Foul odor, usually from axillary vault

PHYSICAL EXAMINATION
- Appearance of skin normal except when associated w/ other unrelated conditions, such as erythrasma or intertrigo

DIFFERENTIAL DIAGNOSIS
- Body dysmorphic disorder
- Fish odor syndrome (trimethylaminuria)
- Organic brain lesions (tumors, etc.)

LABORATORY WORK-UP
- None

MANAGEMENT
- Hygienic measures
- Surgical ablation of apocrine glands

SPECIFIC THERAPY
- Hygienic measures
  - ➤ Adequate washing of axillary vault
  - ➤ Frequent clothing changes
  - ➤ Zeasorb powder applied BID
  - ➤ Dietary changes, including omission of certain foods (e.g., certain spices, garlic, alcohol) when contributory
- Surgical
  - ➤ Superficial liposuction to remove apocrine glands
  - ➤ Excision of axillary vault skin

CAVEATS AND PITFALLS
- None

BULLOUS PEMPHIGOID

ALTERNATE DISEASE NAME
- Pemphigoid
- Pemphigus vulgaris chronicus
- Pemphigoid vegetans

HISTORY
- More common in elderly pts
- May have either gradual or explosive onset
- No effect on general health in most cases

PHYSICAL EXAMINATION
- Tense vesicles & bullae, w/ a predilection for flexor areas
- Lesions may be urticarial without vesiculation
- May have either inflammatory or non-inflammatory blisters, which usually heal without scarring or milia formation
- Localized form w/ blisters confined to extremities
- Oral & ocular mucosa involvement seldom occurs

DIFFERENTIAL DIAGNOSIS
- Erythema multiforme
- Cicatricial pemphigoid
- Herpes gestationis
- Linear IgA bullous dermatosis
- Dermatitis herpetiformis
- Chronic bullous dermatosis of childhood
- Dyshidrosis
- Bullous lupus erythematosus
- Pemphigus vegetans
- Urticaria

LABORATORY WORK-UP
- Diagnostic skin biopsy for routine light microscopy
- Skin biopsy for direct immunofluorescence if diagnosis is in doubt
- Serum for indirect immunofluorescence if diagnosis is in doubt or if biopsy cannot be obtained

MANAGEMENT
- Topical corticosteroids
- Systemic corticosteroids
- Nonsteroidal anti-inflammatory agents
- Systemic steroid-sparing agents

SPECIFIC THERAPY
- Mild to moderate disease
  - High-potency topical corticosteroids, such as clobetasol 0.05% cream applied BID
  - Combination of tetracycline & niacinamide 500 mg PO 2 or 3 times daily
- Severe disease

➤ Prednisone 1 mg/kg PO QAM
➤ Steroid-sparing agents
  • Azathioprine 2–3 mg/kg PO QD
  • Mycophenolate mofetil 1–1.5 g PO BID
  • Dapsone 50–200 mg PO QD
  • Methotrexate 7.5–15 mg PO Q 7 days; caution in those w/ liver disease
  • Cyclophosphamide 100–200 mg PO QD

CAVEATS AND PITFALLS
■ Check thiopurine methyltransferase levels before starting azathioprine therapy.
■ Check CBC every 2–3 wks for 10–12 wks w/ dapsone to detect rare pancytopenia.
■ Use systemic corticosteroids only if less aggressive therapies fail, particularly in elderly pts.

BURNING MOUTH SYNDROME

ALTERNATE DISEASE NAME
■ Orodynia

HISTORY
■ Sensation of pain or burning in the mouth
■ Secondary causes include xerostomia, ill-fitting dentures, vitamin deficiency & contact dermatitis
■ Women more commonly affected

PHYSICAL EXAMINATION
■ Burning pain affecting oropharynx, without evident lesions
■ Onset often in the morning, w/ peak symptoms in late afternoon
■ Lower lip mucosa, anterior tongue, anterior hard palate affected
■ Pain relief w/ eating
■ Associated w/ dry mouth & taste disturbance

DIFFERENTIAL DIAGNOSIS
■ Tobacco abuse
■ Atrophic glossitis
■ Menopausal glossitis
■ Heavy metal poisoning

- Vitamin deficiency
- Lichen planus
- Medication reaction

LABORATORY WORK-UP
- Serum vitamin levels if deficiency is a possibility

MANAGEMENT
- Topical counterirritants
- Tricyclic antidepressants
- Gabapentin
- SSRI agents

SPECIFIC THERAPY
- Capsaicin: starting w/ hot pepper diluted 1:2 w/ water; rinsing of mouth w/ 1 teaspoon; or decreasing dilution to 1:1 as tolerated
- Amitriptyline 25–100 PO QD
- Gabapentin 300 mg PO QD; titrate up to max of 1,800 mg per day
- Celexa 20 mg PO QD

CAVEATS AND PITFALLS
- May be associated w/ signs & symptoms of depression in some pts.

CAFÉ AU LAIT MACULE

ALTERNATE DISEASE NAME
- Café-au-lait spot
- Hypermelanotic macule
- Circumscribed melanotic macule
- Circumscribed hypermelanosis

HISTORY
- Often present at birth
- Most have no associated abnormality
- May occur in pts w/ neurofibromatosis, McCune-Albright syndrome, Watson's syndrome, proteus syndrome, Bloom's syndrome, piebaldism, Fanconi's anemia

PHYSICAL EXAMINATION
- Asymptomatic, 2- to 20-mm discrete tan-brown macule or patch
- May have irregular borders

DIFFERENTIAL DIAGNOSIS
- Lentigo
- Seborrheic keratosis
- Nevocellular nevus
- Nevus spilus
- Multiple lentigines syndrome

LABORATORY WORK-UP
- None

MANAGEMENT
- Laser ablation
- Hydroquinone

SPECIFIC THERAPY
- Q-switched Nd:YAG or Q-switched ruby laser ablation
- Hydroquinone 4% cream or gel applied BID for months; advise about incomplete response in most cases

CAVEATS AND PITFALLS
- Incomplete removal common after any medical or surgical therapy.

CALCINOSIS CUTIS

ALTERNATE DISEASE NAME
- Cutaneous calcification
- Cutaneous calcinosis
- Cutaneous calculi

HISTORY
- Metastatic type
  - ➤ Occurs in chronic renal failure, sarcoidosis, milk-alkali syndrome, hyperparathyroidism & certain neoplastic diseases
  - ➤ May appear after chronic overuse of vitamin D
- Dystrophic type
  - ➤ Occurs in pts w/ rheumatic diseases, such as juvenile dermatomyositis
  - ➤ May appear after local trauma or parasitic infection

- Idiopathic type
  - No obvious antecedent cause of localized calcification

PHYSICAL EXAMINATION
- Multiple, asymptomatic, firm, whitish papules, plaques or nodules in dermis and/or subcutis
- May spontaneously ulcerate & extrude a chalky white material
- Dystrophic calcinosis cutis: deposits at site of trauma
- Metastatic calcification: widespread calcinosis, often around large joints

DIFFERENTIAL DIAGNOSIS
- Gouty tophus
- Foreign body granuloma
- Granuloma annulare
- Xanthoma
- Milium
- Osteoma cutis

LABORATORY WORK-UP
- Serum levels of calcium & phosphate
- Parathyroid hormone level
- Vitamin D_3 level
- 24-hour urine calcium excretion

MANAGEMENT
- Surgical excision
- Calcium channel blockers
- Intralesional corticosteroids

SPECIFIC THERAPY
- Surgical excision
  - Elliptical excision
  - Incision & drainage
- Diltiazem 120–240 mg PO QD
- Triamcinolone 3–4 mg/mL intralesional

CAVEATS AND PITFALLS
- None

CAPILLARY HEMANGIOMA

ALTERNATE DISEASE NAME
- Infantile hemangioma
- Strawberry hemangioma
- Strawberry mark
- Raspberry lesion
- Capillary angioma

HISTORY
- Most common tumor of infancy
- Appears in first several wks of life in most cases
- More common in females

PHYSICAL EXAMINATION
- Early lesion (up to 6 wks of age)
  - Blanching of involved skin w/ telangiectasias
  - Red or violaceous macule or papule, often surrounded by a faint hypopigmented halo
- Proliferative stage (up to 12 months)
  - Dome-shaped, multilobular papule or nodule, which may develop central erosion or ulceration
  - Firm, rubbery consistency, which expands w/ increased intravascular pressure
- Involution stage
  - Tumor shrinks from the center
  - Lesion becomes less red, w/ a dusky maroon to purple color, & regains normal flesh tones ("graying")
- Cavernous variant
  - Deep dermal & subcutaneous red to violaceous nodule
  - Less likely to completely regress

DIFFERENTIAL DIAGNOSIS
- Nevus flammeus or other arteriovenous malformation
- Lymphatic malformation
- Blue rubber bleb syndrome
- Pseudo-Kaposi's hemangioendothelioma
- Mafucci syndrome
- Angiosarcoma

- Infantile fibrosarcoma
- Infantile myofibromatosis
- Teratoma
- Gorham syndrome
- Riley-Smith syndrome

LABORATORY WORK-UP
- None

MANAGEMENT
- No therapy if asymptomatic & not in anatomically sensitive area
- Laser ablation
- Systemic corticosteroids

SPECIFIC THERAPY
- Ulcerated hemangiomas & thin superficial hemangiomas
  - ➤ Flash lamp-pumped pulsed dye laser
- Lesions compromising function (eg, larynx or eyelid)
  - ➤ Prednisolone 2–5 mg/kg per day PO; caution: growth retardation, cataracts & other steroid side effects may occur

CAVEATS AND PITFALLS
- Treatment emergency if lesion threatens to close eye or interferes w/ eating.

CELLULITIS

ALTERNATE DISEASE NAME
- None

HISTORY
- Break in the skin is often entry point for infection
- Prodrome of fever, chills, malaise
- Causative organism is immunocompetent adults is usually *S pyogenes* or *S aureus*

PHYSICAL EXAMINATION
- Four signs of infection: erythema, pain, swelling & warmth, w/ poorly demarcated margins
- Areas of edema & erythema blending into surrounding normal skin
- Signs of lymphangitis & regional lymphadenopathy

DIFFERENTIAL DIAGNOSIS
- Erysipelas
- Stasis dermatitis
- Contact dermatitis
- Arthropod envenomation
- Burn
- Septic arthritis
- Panniculitis

LABORATORY WORK-UP
- Blood cultures

MANAGEMENT
- Hospitalization if signs of systemic toxicity
- Systemic antibiotics

SPECIFIC THERAPY
- Oral antibiotics
  - Dicloxacillin
    - Adults: 250–500 mg PO QID for 10 days
    - Children: 25–50 mg/kg PO QID for 7–10 days
  - Cephalexin
    - Adults: 250–500 mg PO QID for 7–10 days
    - Children: 25–100 mg/kg per day, divided into 4 doses for 7–10 days
  - Azithromycin
    - Adults & children >45 kg: 500 mg PO QD for 3 days
    - Children: Not indicated in those <45 kg in weight
  - Clarithromycin
    - Adults: 250 mg PO twice per day for 5–7 days
    - Children >45 kg: 7.5 mg/kg PO twice per day for 5–7 days; not indicated for those <45 kg in weight
- Systemic antibiotics
  - Nafcillin
    - Adults: 0.5–1.5 g IV q4h for 3–7 days
    - Children: 10–20 mg/kg IV q4h for 3–7 days
  - Cefotaxime
    - Adults: 1 g IV q12h for 3–7 days
    - Children: 12.5–45 mg/kg IV q6h for 3–7 days

CAVEATS AND PITFALLS
- Look for evidence of deeper infection (eg, necrotizing fasciitis) if there is extreme systemic toxicity.
- Recurrence common after infection in chronically edematous lower extremity.

CERCARIAL DERMATITIS

ALTERNATE DISEASE NAME
- Swimmer's itch
- Bather's itch
- Clam digger's itch
- Silt itch
- Swamp itch
- Sedge pool itch

HISTORY
- Occurs after contact w/ animal schistosome larvae in lakes & rivers, often populated by ducks
- Peak incidence in early & mid-summer

PHYSICAL EXAMINATION
- Localized pruritus followed by red macules & papules
- Appears mainly in exposed parts of skin, particularly distal lower extremities
- Inflammatory response peaks at 2–3 days & subsides in 1–2 wks

DIFFERENTIAL DIAGNOSIS
- Creeping eruption
- Seabather's eruption
- Insect bite reaction
- Harvest mite infestation

LABORATORY WORK-UP
- None

MANAGEMENT
- Ice compresses applied for 15–20 minutes 2–4 times per day
- Systemic antihistamines for night-time sedation

SPECIFIC THERAPY
- Self-limited process without therapy

CAVEATS AND PITFALLS
- None

CHANCROID

ALTERNATE DISEASE NAME
- Soft chancre

HISTORY
- Spread by sexual contact
- Caused by gram-negative bacillus *Haemophilus ducreyi*

PHYSICAL EXAMINATION
- Disease in men
  - Constitutional symptoms such as malaise & low-grade fever
  - Painful, erythematous papules at the site of recent sexual contact; evolve into pustules & ulcerations
  - Foreskin most common site of infection, but occasionally appears on shaft, glans, or meatus of penis
  - Regional lymphadenopathy
- Disease in women
  - Ulcers most commonly occur on labia majora but may also appear on labia minora, thigh, perineum or cervix
  - Lesions usually less symptomatic than in men

DIFFERENTIAL DIAGNOSIS
- Syphilis
- Herpes simplex virus infection
- Lymphogranuloma venereum
- Traumatic ulceration
- Aphthae, w/ or w/out Behçet's disease
- Crohn's disease
- Fixed drug reaction

LABORATORY WORK-UP
- Smear of ulcer base or aspirate for Gram stain
- Culture of aspirate

MANAGEMENT
- Systemic antibiotics

SPECIFIC THERAPY
- Azithromycin 1 g PO for 1 dose
- Ciprofloxacin 500 mg PO BID for 3 days
- Ceftriaxone 250 mg IM for 1 dose

CAVEATS AND PITFALLS
- Check for evidence of other sexually transmitted disease, such as chlamydial infection & gonorrhea.

CHEILITIS GRANULOMATOSA

ALTERNATE DISEASE NAME
- Orofacial granulomatosis
- Miescher's granulomatosis
- Miescher-Melkersson-Rosenthal syndrome
- Granulomatous cheilitis
- Miescher's cheilitis granulomatosa

HISTORY
- Most common in young adults in otherwise good health

PHYSICAL EXAMINATION
- First episode of edema of lip
  - Resolves completely in hours or days
  - No constitutional symptoms or signs
- After recurrent episodes of lip edema
  - Recurrences common from days to years, w/ cracking & fissuring in affected lip
  - Occasional constitutional symptoms w/ attacks
  - Slow regression over several years

DIFFERENTIAL DIAGNOSIS
- Angioedema
- Lip trauma
- Sarcoidosis
- Dental abscess
- Insect bite reaction
- Crohn's disease

LABORATORY WORK-UP
- Lip biopsy only if diagnosis is in doubt

MANAGEMENT
- Intralesional corticosteroids
- Surgical debulking

SPECIFIC THERAPY
- Triamcinolone 3–4 mg/mL intralesional
- Surgical debulking of lip tissue

CAVEATS AND PITFALLS
- Lip swelling may persist permanently if present for many months.

CHERRY HEMANGIOMA

ALTERNATE DISEASE NAME
- Cherry angioma
- Senile angioma
- Campbell de Morgan spots

HISTORY
- Onset usually in middle age
- Increased number of lesions & size w/ advancing age

PHYSICAL EXAMINATION
- Small, red to violaceous macule or a larger dome-shaped or polypoid papule
- May occur on all body sites except mucous membranes

DIFFERENTIAL DIAGNOSIS
- Angiokeratoma
- Petechiae
- Kaposi's sarcoma
- Bacillary angiomatosis
- Vasculitis
- Benign pigmented purpura
- Insect bite reaction
- Blue rubber bleb syndrome

LABORATORY WORK-UP
- None

MANAGEMENT
- Destructive modality, only for cosmetic purposes

SPECIFIC THERAPY
- Destruction by electrodesiccation & curettage
- Liquid nitrogen cryotherapy
- Pulse dye laser ablation

CAVEATS AND PITFALLS
- Scarring may ensue after destructive procedure.

CHILBLAINS

ALTERNATE DISEASE NAME
- Pernio
- Perniosis

HISTORY
- Occurs in predisposed pts who are exposed to cold, damp climates
- Most common in women, children or the elderly
- May occur in association w/ systemic diseases, including chronic myelomonocytic leukemia, anorexia nervosa, dysproteinemias, macroglobulinemia, cryoglobulinemia, cryofibrinogenemia, antiphospholipid antibody syndrome or Raynaud disease

PHYSICAL EXAMINATION
- Appears 12–24 hours after cold exposure
- Recurrent, painful and/or pruritic, red to violaceous papules or nodules on fingers and/or toes
- May produce vesicles or shallow ulcerations

DIFFERENTIAL DIAGNOSIS
- Raynaud phenomenon
- Erythromelalgia
- Vasculitis

- Sarcoidosis
- Erythema multiforme
- Acrocyanosis
- Septic or cholesterol emboli
- Polycythemia vera
- Coumadin-induced purple toe syndrome

LABORATORY WORK-UP
- Consider autoimmune laboratory profile if there are other supporting signs & symptoms

MANAGEMENT
- Prophylactic warming of acral areas w/ minimization of cold exposure
- Calcium channel blockers

SPECIFIC THERAPY
- Nifedipine 20–60 mg PO QD

CAVEATS AND PITFALLS
- None

CHONDRODERMATITIS NODULARIS

ALTERNATE DISEASE NAME
- Chondrodermatitis nodularis chronica helicis
- Chondrodermatitis nodularis chronica antihelicis

HISTORY
- Painful lesion on ear
- Occurs mainly in those who put recurrent pressure on the site, such as chronic telephone over-users

PHYSICAL EXAMINATION
- Firm, tender, well-demarcated papule w/ a raised, rolled edge & central erosion or ulceration
- Appears on the most prominent projection of the ear, most commonly on the apex of the helix
- Distribution on the antihelix more common in women

DIFFERENTIAL DIAGNOSIS
- Squamous cell carcinoma

- Actinic keratosis
- Basal cell carcinoma
- Keratoacanthoma
- Gouty tophus
- Rheumatoid nodule
- Colloid milium
- Endochondral pseudocyst

LABORATORY WORK-UP
- Diagnostic skin biopsy

MANAGEMENT
- Remove source of pressure at site of involvement
  - ➤ Use speakerphone instead of hand-held device
  - ➤ Specially designed pillow for sleeping (CHN pillow)
- Destructive modality
- Excision

SPECIFIC THERAPY
- Elliptical excision, including underlying cartilage
- Destructive modalities
  - ➤ Cryotherapy
  - ➤ Triamcinolone 3–5 mg/mL intralesional

CAVEATS AND PITFALLS
- Often looks exactly like basal cell carcinoma; diagnostic biopsy before therapy if any question.

CHROMOMYCOSIS

ALTERNATE DISEASE NAME
- Chromoblastomycosis
- Verrucous dermatitis
- Phaeohyphomycosis
- Cystic chromomycosis

HISTORY
- Caused by several genera of pigmented fungi
- Most commonly found in rural areas in tropical climates, in men as a result of occupational exposure

PHYSICAL EXAMINATION
- Asymptomatic, verrucous papule, slowly enlarging to large plaque or thick nodule, which may ulcerate
- Satellite lesions produced by autoinoculation

DIFFERENTIAL DIAGNOSIS
- South American blastomycosis
- North American blastomycosis
- Atypical mycobacterial infection
- Sporotrichosis
- Nocardiosis
- Tuberculosis
- Leishmaniasis
- Syphilis
- Yaws
- Squamous cell carcinoma

LABORATORY WORK-UP
- Biopsy for routine histology & culture

MANAGEMENT
- Localized hyperthermia
- Systemic antifungal antibiotics
- Destructive modalities

SPECIFIC THERAPY
- Itraconazole 200 mg twice per day 1 wk per month for 7 months
- Terbinafine 250 mg PO per day for 3–6 months

CAVEATS AND PITFALLS
- Chronic infection often never heals completely.

CHRONIC ACTINIC DERMATITIS

ALTERNATE DISEASE NAME
- Actinic reticuloid
- Persistent light reactivity
- Photosensitive eczema
- Photosensitivity dermatitis

HISTORY
- Chronic, recurrent eruption following exposure to ultraviolet light & sometimes visible light sources, usually occurring in the elderly
- May be associated w/ airborne contact dermatitis

PHYSICAL EXAMINATION
- Eczematous & infiltrated plaques that initially involve exposed skin
- Occasional generalized erythroderma

DIFFERENTIAL DIAGNOSIS
- Polymorphous light eruption
- Allergic contact dermatitis
- Photocontact dermatitis
- Actinic prurigo
- Atopic dermatitis
- Lupus erythematosus
- Cutaneous T-cell lymphoma
- Solar urticaria

LABORATORY WORK-UP
- Patch testing, including photopatch testing
- Irradiation photo-testing w/ UVB, UVA & visible light
- Skin biopsy for diagnosis confirmation

MANAGEMENT
- Protection from light sources, including visible light
- Protective clothing
- Topical corticosteroids
- Immunosuppressive agents
- Phototherapy

SPECIFIC THERAPY
- Fluocinonide 0.05% cream applied twice daily
- Azathioprine 2–3 mg/kg PO daily
- Cyclosporine 3–5 mg/kg PO daily
- UVB phototherapy
- Photochemotherapy

CAVEATS AND PITFALLS

■ Obtain baseline thiopurine methyltransferase level before starting azathioprine.

■ Closely monitor renal function & blood pressure with cyclosporine therapy.

CICATRICIAL PEMPHIGOID

ALTERNATE DISEASE NAME

■ Benign mucous membrane pemphigoid

■ Scarring pemphigoid

■ Mucosal pemphigoid

HISTORY

■ Most common in the elderly

■ Insidious onset of painful lesions in mucous membranes

PHYSICAL EXAMINATION

■ Ocular involvement
  ➤ Pain or sensation of grittiness in the eye
  ➤ Conjunctival inflammation & erosions
  ➤ Keratinization of conjunctiva & shortening of fornices
  ➤ May develop entropion w/ subsequent trichiasis

■ Skin
  ➤ Tense vesicles or bullae, sometimes hemorrhagic
  ➤ Lesions often heal w/ scarring or milia
  ➤ Scalp involvement sometimes causes alopecia

DIFFERENTIAL DIAGNOSIS

■ Bullous pemphigoid

■ Linear IgA dermatosis

■ Erythema multiforme

■ Stevens-Johnson syndrome

■ Epidermolysis bullosa

■ Epidermolysis bullosa acquisita

■ Dermatitis herpetiformis

■ Impetigo

■ Pemphigus foliaceous

■ Pemphigus vulgaris

- Herpes simplex virus infection
- Herpes zoster

LABORATORY WORK-UP
- Skin and/or mucous membrane biopsy for routine histology
- Skin and/or mucous membrane biopsy for direct immunofluorescence if diagnosis is in doubt after routine histology

MANAGEMENT
- Topical corticosteroids for mild disease
- Systemic corticosteroids
- Systemic corticosteroid-sparing agents
- Surgical correction of ocular anatomic defects

SPECIFIC THERAPY
- Limited disease
  - Fluocinonide 0.05% gel applied 3 or 4 times daily to mucous membranes
- Extensive disease
  - Prednisone 1–2 mg/kg PO QAM
  - Corticosteroid-sparing agents
    - Dapsone 50–150 mg PO QD
    - Cyclophosphamide 1–2 mg/kg PO QD
    - Azathioprine 2–3 mg/kg PO QD

CAVEATS AND PITFALLS
- If prednisone is to be used for >21 days per course of therapy, obtain baseline chest radiograph, TB skin test & bone mineral density determination.
- Check CBC every 2–3 wks for 10–12 wks w/ dapsone to detect rare pancytopenia.
- Obtain baseline thiopurine methyltransferase level before starting azathioprine.
- Closely monitor renal function & blood pressure w/ cyclosporine therapy.

CLAVUS

ALTERNATE DISEASE NAME
- Callus

- Callous
- Callosity
- Corn
- Heloma

HISTORY
- Bony abnormalities often are under area of involvement
- Repeated frictional trauma is proximate cause

PHYSICAL EXAMINATION
- Thickened skin, w/ retained skin dermatoglyphics, most commonly on the foot
- Occasional secondary maceration & fungal or bacterial infection

DIFFERENTIAL DIAGNOSIS
- Wart
- Lichen simplex chronicus
- Palmoplantar keratoderma
- Porokeratosis plantaris
- Gouty tophus
- Lichen planus
- Interdigital neuroma

LABORATORY WORK-UP
- None

MANAGEMENT
- Mechanical pressure redistribution

SPECIFIC THERAPY
- Mechanical pressure redistribution
  - Orthotics
  - Well-fitted shoes
  - Protective pads on pressure points
- Skin-surface paring only for symptomatic lesions

CAVEATS AND PITFALLS
- Do not pare asymptomatic calluses, especially in athletes w/ sports-related callosities.

COCCIDIOIDOMYCOSIS, DISSEMINATED

ALTERNATE DISEASE NAME
- Valley fever
- San Joaquin Valley fever
- Desert rheumatism
- Coccidiosis

HISTORY
- Endemic in southwest USA, central California, northern Mexico, Central & South America
- Caused by dimorphic fungal pathogen *C. immitis*, usually inhaled in dust

PHYSICAL EXAMINATION
- Skin disease almost always indicates dissemination
- Prodrome of fever, weight loss, malaise & headache
- Acute or subacute pneumonic illness most common clinical presentation, w/ cough & inspiratory chest pain
- Specific skin findings
  - Superficial red, firm papules
  - Keratotic nodules
  - Verrucous ulcers
  - Subcutaneous fluctuant abscesses
  - Other organs of dissemination include bones & joints, adrenal glands, CNS & liver
- Nonspecific skin findings
  - Erythema nodosum
  - Erythema multiforme

DIFFERENTIAL DIAGNOSIS
- Rosacea
- Tinea faciei
- Tuberculosis
- Sarcoidosis
- Actinomycosis
- Sporotrichosis
- Chromomycosis
- Leishmaniasis
- Wegener's granulomatosis

- Cutaneous vasculitis
- Syphilis
- Mycosis fungoides
- Lichen planus

LABORATORY WORK-UP
- Chest radiograph
- Serologies for coccidioidomycosis
- Lesional biopsy for light microscopy & fungal culture

MANAGEMENT
- Systemic antifungal antibiotics

SPECIFIC THERAPY
- Amphotericin B
  - First-line therapy for life-threatening disease
  - 0.3–1 mg/kg per day IV; start with 0.25 mg/kg per day & increase by 5–10 mg per day
- Fluconazole 200–400 mg PO QD for at least 6 months
- Itraconazole 200 mg PO BID for at least 6 months

CAVEATS AND PITFALLS
- Increased concern for dissemination in blacks & Filipinos.
- Recurrences more likely if pt becomes immunosuppressed.

COLD PANNICULITIS

ALTERNATE DISEASE NAME
- Popsicle panniculitis
- Haxthausen's disease

HISTORY
- Occurs 1–3 days after cold exposure, such as popsicle ingestion

PHYSICAL EXAMINATION
- Occurs on exposed or poorly protected areas of skin
- Painful, firm, red or cyanotic, indurated nodules w/ ill-defined margins
- In obese pts, buttocks, thighs, arms & area under the chin are most commonly affected sites
- In small children, most common site of involvement is cheeks

DIFFERENTIAL DIAGNOSIS
- Subcutaneous fat necrosis of the newborn
- Sclerema neonatorum
- Cellulitis
- Post-steroid panniculitis
- Erythema infectiosum
- Atopic dermatitis

LABORATORY WORK-UP
- None

MANAGEMENT
- Self-limited process, requiring no therapy

SPECIFIC THERAPY
- None

CAVEATS AND PITFALLS
- None

CONDYLOMA ACUMINATUM

ALTERNATE DISEASE NAME
- Genital wart
- Anogenital wart
- Condyloma acuminata

HISTORY
- Occurs mainly but not exclusively in sexually active individuals
- May be sign of child abuse
- May be severe in immunocompromised pts

PHYSICAL EXAMINATION
- Pink to brown, verrucous, soft papules or nodules of the genitalia, perineum, crural folds & anus
- May form large, exophytic, cauliflower-like tumors

DIFFERENTIAL DIAGNOSIS
- Seborrheic keratosis
- Pearly penile papules
- Syphilis

- Verrucous carcinoma of genitalia (giant condyloma of Buschke-Löwenstein)
- Bowenoid papulosis
- Anogenital carcinoma
- Erythroplasia of Queyrat
- Lichen planus
- Reiter syndrome

LABORATORY WORK-UP
- None

MANAGEMENT
- Destructive modalities
- Topical keratolytic or antiviral agents
- Surgical excision or debulking of large tumors

SPECIFIC THERAPY
- Destructive modalities
  - Cryotherapy
  - Destruction by electrodesiccation & curettage
  - CO_2 laser ablation
- Topical agents
  - Imiquimod applied TIW
  - Podofilox applied BID for 3 consecutive days per week for up to 4 weeks

CAVEATS AND PITFALLS
- Advise about irritation w/ imiquimod & podofilox therapy.
- Anoscopy indicated in all perianal warts because of possibility of intrarectal lesions.

CONGENITAL ERYTHROPOIETIC PORPHYRIA

ALTERNATE DISEASE NAME
- Günther's disease
- Erythropoietic porphyria
- Congenital porphyria
- Porphyria erythropoietica
- Congenital hematoporphyria
- Erythropoietic uroporphyria

HISTORY
- Familial clustering
- Severe photosensitivity from birth

PHYSICAL EXAMINATION
- Blistering & fragility of light-exposed skin
- Hypertrichosis
- Reddish hue in teeth
- Eye changes
  - Blepharitis
  - Cicatricial ectropion
  - Conjunctivitis
- Secondary hypersplenism

DIFFERENTIAL DIAGNOSIS
- Erythropoietic protoporphyria
- Polymorphous light eruption
- Porphyria cutanea tarda
- Xeroderma pigmentosum
- Bloom's syndrome
- Variegate porphyria

LABORATORY WORK-UP
- Urine for uroporphyrin & coproporphyrin
- Stool for coproporphyrin
- Blood sample for RBC uroporphyrin, protoporphyrin & coproporphyrin

MANAGEMENT
- Strict sun avoidance
- Splenectomy for hemolytic anemia
- Bone marrow transplantation
- Porphyrin binding agents

SPECIFIC THERAPY
- Erythrocyte transfusion to suppress erythropoiesis
- Beta-carotene 120–300 mg PO QD
- Porphyrin binding agents
  - Activated charcoal 60 g PO TID

CAVEATS AND PITFALLS
- None

CONNECTIVE TISSUE NEVUS

ALTERNATE DISEASE NAME
- Collagenoma
- Elastoma
- Nevus mucinosis

HISTORY
- Usually present at birth or arises in early childhood

PHYSICAL EXAMINATION
- Multiple, indurated, cutaneous papules or nodules, often over upper two thirds of the back
- Associated w/ multiple endocrine neoplasia (MEN) type I
- Shagreen patch: connective tissue nevus in a pt w/ tuberous sclerosis
- Nevus mucinosis (Hunter syndrome)
  - Small, firm papules on arms & chest & over scapular region
  - Associated w/ coarse facial features, mental retardation & deafness

DIFFERENTIAL DIAGNOSIS
- Milia
- Morphea
- Scar
- Athlete's nodules (knuckle pads, etc.)
- Cowden disease

LABORATORY WORK-UP
- Skin biopsy only if diagnosis is in doubt

MANAGEMENT
- Surgical excision

SPECIFIC THERAPY
- Surgical excision for cosmetic reasons only

CAVEATS AND PITFALLS
- Common recurrences w/ incomplete excision.

CONTACT DERMATITIS

ALTERNATE DISEASE NAME
- Contact eczema
- Dermatitis venenata

HISTORY
- Eruption begins 48–72 hours after contact w/ suspect antigen

PHYSICAL EXAMINATION
- Acute contact stage
  - Red & edematous skin
  - Vesicles or bullae after extreme inflammation
  - Weeping & oozing as vesicles rupture
- Subacute stage
  - Less edematous & erythematous than acute stage
  - Scaling & punctate crusts from scratching
- Chronic stage: scaling, fissuring & lichenification w/ minimal edema
- Contact urticaria variant: urticarial wheals at site of contact
- Phototoxic variant: appearance of an exaggerated sunburn

DIFFERENTIAL DIAGNOSIS
- Atopic dermatitis
- Dyshidrotic eczema
- Chemical burn
- Seborrheic dermatitis
- Erysipelas
- Erythema multiforme
- Nummular eczema
- Asteatotic eczema
- Sunburn
- Bullous pemphigoid
- Pemphigus vulgaris
- Epidermolysis bullosa
- Dermatophyte infection
- Candidiasis
- Impetigo
- Scabies
- Insect bites

LABORATORY WORK-UP
- Patch testing for suspect antigens

MANAGEMENT
- Remove source of dermatitis
- Topical and/or systemic corticosteroids

SPECIFIC THERAPY
- Mild to moderate disease
  - Topical corticosteroids
    - Triamcinolone 0.1% cream applied BID
    - Fluocinonide 0.05% cream applied BID
  - Aluminum acetate 5% compresses applied 15–30 minutes 2–4 times daily
- Severe disease
  - Prednisone 1 mg/kg PO QD for 7–14 days
  - Diphenhydramine 50 mg PO HS or doxepin 25 mg PO HS for sedation

CAVEATS AND PITFALLS
- Use prednisone for a maximum of 21 days.

COUMARIN NECROSIS

ALTERNATE DISEASE NAME
- Coumarin skin necrosis
- Warfarin skin necrosis

HISTORY
- Acquired transient protein C dysfunction
- Occurs after 2–5 days of coumadin therapy
- Most common after loading doses of coumadin w/out heparin anticoagulation

PHYSICAL EXAMINATION
- Single or multiple areas of painful erythema, rapidly ulcerating & developing a blue-black eschar
- Most common areas of involvement include thighs, breasts & buttocks

DIFFERENTIAL DIAGNOSIS
- Other coagulopathies
- Heparin necrosis
- Necrotizing soft tissue infection
- Spider bite reaction
- Pyoderma gangrenosum
- Vasculitis
- Cutaneous anthrax
- Traumatic ulceration
- Calciphylaxis

LABORATORY WORK-UP
- Protein C level
- Skin biopsy

MANAGEMENT
- Continue coumarin therapy
- Hydrocolloid dressings
- Skin grafting only after delayed healing

SPECIFIC THERAPY
- See "Management"

CAVEATS AND PITFALLS
- Severe scarring at site of involvement is expected.

CRYOGLOBULINEMIA

ALTERNATE DISEASE NAME
- Cryoproteinemia

HISTORY
- Often associated w/ autoimmune diseases such as SLE & rheumatoid arthritis, mycoplasma pneumonia, viral hepatitis, myeloma & leukemia
- Acute & paroxysmal constitutional signs & symptoms

PHYSICAL EXAMINATION
- Skin findings
  - ➤ Palpable purpura, in retiform pattern
  - ➤ Urticarial papules & plaques, often cold-induced

➤ Ischemic necrosis leading to ulceration
➤ Acrocyanosis
- Internal manifestations include involvement of lungs, kidneys, CNS & joints

DIFFERENTIAL DIAGNOSIS
- Antiphospholipid antibody syndrome
- Septic vasculitis
- Polyarteritis nodosa
- Serum sickness
- Waldenström hyperglobulinemia
- Sarcoidosis
- Churg-Strauss syndrome
- Chilblains

LABORATORY WORK-UP
- Serum cryoglobulin level
- Skin biopsy

MANAGEMENT
- Minimize cold exposure
- No therapy indicated for asymptomatic disease
- Nonsteroidal anti-inflammatory agents
- Systemic corticosteroids
- Corticosteroid-sparing agents

SPECIFIC THERAPY
- Prednisone 1 mg/kg PO QAM
- Steroid-sparing agents
  ➤ Azathioprine 2–3 mg/kg PO QD; check thiopurine methyl-transferase levels at baseline
  ➤ Mycophenolate mofetil 1–1.5 g PO BID
  ➤ Dapsone 50–200 mg PO QD; check CBC Q2–3 weeks for first 12 weeks
  ➤ Methotrexate 7.5–15 mg PO Q 7 days; caution in pts w/ liver disease
  ➤ Cyclophosphamide 100–200 mg PO QD

CAVEATS AND PITFALLS
- If prednisone is to be used for >21 days per course of therapy, obtain baseline chest radiograph, TB skin test & bone mineral density determination.

- Check CBC Q2–3 weeks for 10–12 weeks w/ dapsone to detect rare pancytopenia.
- Obtain baseline thiopurine methyltransferase level before starting azathioprine.
- Closely monitor renal function & blood pressure w/ cyclosporine therapy.

CUTIS LAXA

ALTERNATE DISEASE NAME
- Cutis pendula
- Dermatochalasis
- Elastolysis
- Dermatomegaly
- Elastolysis cutis laxa

HISTORY
- Presents at birth & progresses throughout life

PHYSICAL EXAMINATION
- Skin loose, inelastic, hanging in folds, w/ decreased elastic recoil on stretching
- Appears much older than chronologic age
- Internal organ involvement
  - GI tract: diverticula of small & large bowel, rectal prolapse, umbilical, inguinal & hiatal hernias
  - Pulmonary: bronchiectasis, emphysema, cor pulmonale
  - Cardiovascular: cardiomegaly, congestive heart failure, murmurs, aortic aneurysms
  - Musculoskeletal: dislocation of hips, osteoporosis, growth retardation, delayed fontanelle closure, ligamentous laxity

DIFFERENTIAL DIAGNOSIS
- Ehlers-Danlos syndrome
- Marfan syndrome
- Granulomatous slack skin variant of peripheral T-cell lymphoma
- Mid-dermal elastolysis
- Pseudoxanthoma elasticum
- Anetoderma

■ Atrophoderma of Pasini & Pierini
■ Costello syndrome

LABORATORY WORK-UP
■ None

MANAGEMENT
■ Reconstructive surgery

SPECIFIC THERAPY
■ See "Management"

CAVEATS AND PITFALLS
■ Results of reconstructive surgery are not permanent.

CUTIS VERTICIS GYRATA

ALTERNATE DISEASE NAME
■ Cutis verticis plicata
■ Robert-Unna syndrome
■ Bulldog scalp
■ Cutis sulcata
■ Corrugated skin
■ Pachydermia verticis gyrata

HISTORY
■ May occur at or near birth (secondary form) or at puberty & beyond (primary form)

PHYSICAL EXAMINATION
■ Limited to scalp
■ Symmetrical, soft & spongy folds, usually in vertex & occipital region
■ Hair over the folds is sometimes sparse, but normal in the furrows
■ Maceration & unpleasant odor may be present in pts w/ secondary infections in the furrows

DIFFERENTIAL DIAGNOSIS
■ Congenital nevus
■ Acromegaly
■ Cutis laxa

- Pachydermoperiostosis
- Cylindroma

LABORATORY WORK-UP
- None

MANAGEMENT
- Surgical resection only for psychological or esthetic reasons

SPECIFIC THERAPY
- See "Management"

CAVEATS AND PITFALLS
- None

CYLINDROMA

ALTERNATE DISEASE NAME
- Turban tumor
- Tomato tumor

HISTORY
- Onset usually in adult life
- Family history in pts w/ multiple tumors

PHYSICAL EXAMINATION
- Solitary tumor subtype
  - Firm, rubbery, red to blue papule or nodule, located on scalp, head or neck
  - Rare malignant transformation
- Multiple tumor subtype
  - Numerous masses of pink, red or blue papules or nodules, sometimes resembling bunches of small tomatoes
  - May be located on head & neck region, trunk or extremities

DIFFERENTIAL DIAGNOSIS
- Pilar cyst
- Eccrine spiradenoma
- Basal cell carcinoma
- Cutaneous metastases
- Cutis verticis gyrata

LABORATORY WORK-UP
- Biopsy of lesional skin

MANAGEMENT
- Surgical excision or laser ablation for esthetic reasons

SPECIFIC THERAPY
- Solitary or multiple small tumors
  - Simple excision or CO_2 laser ablation
- Multiple clustered tumors
  - Multiple excisions w/ reconstruction

CAVEATS AND PITFALLS
- None

CYSTICERCOSIS

ALTERNATE DISEASE NAME
- Neurocysticercosis
- *Taenia solium* infestation

HISTORY
- Occurs in Africa, South America & Southeast Asia
- Occurs because of ingestion of inadequately cooked pork

PHYSICAL EXAMINATION
- Cutaneous changes
  - Subcutaneous nodules resembling epidermoid cysts
- Neurologic findings
  - Papilledema and/or decreased retinal venous pulsations
  - Meningismus
  - Hyperreflexia
  - Nystagmus or other visual deficits
- Musculoskeletal findings: muscle pseudohypertrophy

DIFFERENTIAL DIAGNOSIS
- Toxoplasmosis
- CNS tumor
- Tuberculosis
- Meningitis
- Encephalitis
- Brain abscess
- Cerebrovascular accident

- Sarcoidosis
- Coccidioidomycosis

LABORATORY WORK-UP
- Examination of stool & perianal area for eggs

MANAGEMENT
- Surgical excision of solitary lesions
- Systemic anthelminthic therapy

SPECIFIC THERAPY
- Albendazole 15 mg/kg per day PO divided into 2 or 3 doses for 2 weeks
- Praziquantel 50 mg/kg per day PO divided into 3 doses for 2 weeks

CAVEATS AND PITFALLS
- Poor response to medical therapy in many cases.

DARIER DISEASE

ALTERNATE DISEASE NAME
- Darier's disease
- Darier-White disease
- Keratosis follicularis

HISTORY
- Familial clustering
- Peak onset at puberty, but may first appear much later in life
- Heat, humidity, stress, sunlight & UVB rays may worsen the condition
- Appearance & odor may lead to social isolation

PHYSICAL EXAMINATION
- Yellowish-brown, greasy, verrucous papules, most common in seborrheic areas such as forehead, scalp, nasolabial folds, ears, chest & back
- Mucosal surfaces w/ white papules w/ central depression
- Palmar lesions include punctate keratosis, palmar pits & hemorrhagic macules
- Verrucous papules on backs of hands
- Nail changes include white & red longitudinal bands, longitudinal nail ridges & splits

DIFFERENTIAL DIAGNOSIS
- Transient acantholytic dermatosis
- Hailey-Hailey disease
- Pemphigus foliaceus
- Seborrheic dermatitis
- Pityriasis lichenoides chronica
- Folliculitis
- Follicular eczema
- Acrokeratosis verruciformis of Hopf

LABORATORY WORK-UP
- Skin biopsy only if diagnosis is in question

MANAGEMENT
- Systemic & topical retinoids
- Dermabrasion or laser resurfacing for local control
- Genetic counseling

SPECIFIC THERAPY
- Isotretinoin 0.2–0.3 mg/kg PO per day for 1 month, followed by 0.5–1.0 mg/kg per day indefinitely
- Tretinoin 0.025% cream applied HS indefinitely
- Tazarotene 0.1% gel applied QD indefinitely

CAVEATS AND PITFALLS
- Advise about irritation w/ tretinoin & tazarotene therapy.
- Long-term systemic retinoid therapy associated w/ spinal hyperostosis.

DECUBITUS ULCER

ALTERNATE DISEASE NAME
- Pressure ulcer
- Decubitus
- Pressure sore
- Ischemic ulcer
- Bed sore

HISTORY
- Most lesions develop in hospital or nursing home setting

- Risk factors include sensory deficit, prolonged immobilization, poor nutrition & circulatory abnormality

PHYSICAL EXAMINATION
- Stage 1: intact skin w/ signs of impending ulceration, w/ blanching erythema from reactive hyperemia
- Stage 2: partial-thickness loss of skin involving epidermis & some dermis; may begin as an abrasion, blister or superficial ulceration
- Stage 3: full-thickness loss of skin w/ extension into subcutaneous tissue but not through underlying fascia
- Stage 4: full-thickness loss of skin & subcutaneous tissue w/ extension into muscle, bone, tendon or joint capsule

DIFFERENTIAL DIAGNOSIS
- Pyoderma gangrenosum
- Squamous cell carcinoma
- Factitial ulcer
- Envenomation
- Stasis ulcer
- Vasculitis
- Burn or other trauma
- Contact dermatitis
- Bullous pemphigoid

LABORATORY WORK-UP
- Skin biopsy of ulcer edge to rule out squamous cell carcinoma, only in very chronic ulcers

MANAGEMENT
- Reduction or elimination of the source of external pressure, w/ frequent turning, protective pads, special mattresses, etc.
- Stage 2: hydrocolloid dressings
- Stages 3 & 4: wet dressings; hydrogels; xerogels
- Whirlpool debridement

SPECIFIC THERAPY
- None

CAVEATS AND PITFALLS
- Observe for possible secondary bacterial infection in chronic ulceration.

DERMATITIS HERPETIFORMIS

ALTERNATE DISEASE NAME
- Dühring's disease
- Dühring-Bloch disease
- Hydroa herpetiformis
- Pemphigus circinatus

HISTORY
- Usually arises in adult life
- Occasional connection with symptomatic gluten-sensitive enteropathy

PHYSICAL EXAMINATION
- Tense vesicles on an erythematous base, occurring in tight clusters (herpetiform pattern), symmetrically distributed over extensor surfaces, including elbows, knees, buttocks, shoulders & posterior scalp
- Occasional occurrence of erosions & crusts in the absence of vesicles
- Symptoms include burning, stinging & intense pruritus
- Oral mucosa lesions occur infrequently
- Palms & soles usually spared
- GI symptoms usually mild or absent

DIFFERENTIAL DIAGNOSIS
- Bullous pemphigoid
- Erythema multiforme
- Epidermolysis bullosa
- Epidermolysis bullosa acquisita
- Linear IgA dermatosis
- Impetigo
- Pemphigus foliaceous
- Pemphigus vulgaris
- Herpes simplex virus infection
- Herpes zoster

LABORATORY WORK-UP
- Lesional biopsy

■ Skin biopsy of normal perilesional skin for immunofluorescence if diagnosis is in doubt

MANAGEMENT
■ Gluten-free diet
■ Sulfones or sulfapyridine
■ Prednisone

SPECIFIC THERAPY
■ Dapsone 25 to 200 mg PO QD
■ Sulfapyridine 500 to 1,000 mg PO BID
■ Prednisone 0.5 to 1 mg/kg PO QAM

CAVEATS AND PITFALLS
■ Extremely difficult to maintain gluten-free diet.
■ Check CBC Q2–3 weeks for 10–12 weeks w/ dapsone to detect rare pancytopenia.
  ➤ Obtain baseline G6PD level before dapsone therapy.
■ If prednisone is to be used for >21 days per course of therapy, obtain baseline chest radiograph, TB skin test & bone mineral density determination.

DERMATOFIBROMA

ALTERNATE DISEASE NAME
■ Histiocytoma
■ Sclerosing hemangioma
■ Fibroma simplex
■ Dermal dendrocytoma
■ Dermatofibroma lenticulare
■ Histiocytoma cutis
■ Nodular subepidermal fibrosis
■ Sclerosing angioma

HISTORY
■ Occurs mainly on the extremities of adults
■ Multiple lesions suggest hereditary predisposition

PHYSICAL EXAMINATION
■ Solitary, flesh-colored to brown, firm, asymptomatic or mildly tender papule, usually on the extremities

- May have multiple lesions
- Tethering of the overlying epidermis to the underlying lesion w/ lateral compression (dimple or button sign)

DIFFERENTIAL DIAGNOSIS
- Nevocellular nevus
- Seborrheic keratosis
- Scar
- Keloid
- Melanoma
- Basal cell carcinoma
- Dermatofibrosarcoma protuberans
- Wart
- Epidermoid cyst
- Prurigo nodularis
- Desmoplastic trichoepithelioma
- Foreign body granuloma
- Mastocytoma
- Metastasis
- Juvenile xanthogranuloma

LABORATORY WORK-UP
- None

MANAGEMENT
- Surgical excision or destruction for cosmetic reasons only

SPECIFIC THERAPY
- Elliptical excision
- Shave removal
- Destruction by cryotherapy

CAVEATS AND PITFALLS
- Scar after surgery may look worse than original lesion.
- Advise about post-procedure hypopigmentation w/ cryotherapy.

DERMATOFIBROSARCOMA PROTUBERANS

ALTERNATE DISEASE NAME
- Bednar tumor

- Fibrosarcoma of the skin
- Progressive & recurring dermatofibroma
- Hypertrophic morphea

HISTORY
- Slow-growing tumor in young to middle-age adults

PHYSICAL EXAMINATION
- Presents as small, asymptomatic papule, most commonly on trunk or proximal upper extremities
- Gradually enlarges into indurated plaque, composed of firm, irregular nodules, varying from flesh-colored to reddish-brown

DIFFERENTIAL DIAGNOSIS
- Dermatofibroma
- Keloid
- Melanoma
- Morphea
- Cutaneous metastasis
- Lymphoma

LABORATORY WORK-UP
- Skin biopsy

MANAGEMENT
- Excisional surgery

SPECIFIC THERAPY
- Mohs micrographic surgery
- Wide, local excision

CAVEATS AND PITFALLS
- Frequent recurrences after incomplete excision.

DERMATOMYOSITIS, CUTANEOUS

ALTERNATE DISEASE NAME
- Dermatomyositis sine myositis
- Amyopathic dermatomyositis

HISTORY
- Skin disease may be initial or only manifestation

- Muscle disease may precede or follow skin disease by weeks to years
- Eruption may be sun-sensitive
- May be associated w/ underlying malignancy in pts over age 50

PHYSICAL EXAMINATION
- Violaceous to dusky, erythematous plaques w/ or w/out edema in a symmetrical distribution involving periorbital skin & upper eyelids
- Central facial erythema
- Scalp involvement
  - Erythematous-to-violaceous psoriasiform plaques
  - Slightly elevated, violaceous papules & plaques
- Red papules over bony prominences, particularly the metacarpophalangeal joints, proximal interphalangeal joints and/or distal interphalangeal joints (Gottron papules)
- Violaceous, scaly plaques over elbows, knees and/or feet
- Periungual telangiectases
- Irregular, ragged cuticles w/ hypertrophy & hemorrhagic infarcts
- Calcinosis of the skin or muscle common in children or adolescents

DIFFERENTIAL DIAGNOSIS
- Lupus erythematosus
- Psoriasis
- Lichen planus
- Scleroderma
- Seborrheic dermatitis
- Pemphigus foliaceous
- Polymorphous light eruption
- Dermatophytosis
- Parapsoriasis
- Rosacea
- Sarcoidosis

LABORATORY WORK-UP
- Skin biopsy
- Serum CPK, aldolase
- MRI, muscle biopsy, EMG w/ symptomatic muscle disease

■ Evaluation for overlapping rheumatic diseases (e.g., SLE) w/ suggestive signs & symptoms

MANAGEMENT
■ Systemic corticosteroids
■ Corticosteroid-sparing agents
■ Surgical removal of calcium deposits

SPECIFIC THERAPY
■ Prednisone 1 mg/kg PO QAM; switch to alternate-day therapy if possible after clinical response
■ Corticosteroid-sparing drugs
  ➤ Methotrexate 7.5–15 mg/d PO Q 1 week
  ➤ Azathioprine 2–3 mg/kg PO QD
  ➤ Cyclosporine 3–5 mg/kg PO divided into 2 daily doses
  ➤ Cyclophosphamide 50–200 mg PO QD
  ➤ Hydroxychloroquine 200 mg PO BID
  ➤ Mycophenolate mofetil 1–1.5 g PO BID
  ➤ IVIG 1 g IV on 2 successive days, repeated every 4–6 weeks as needed

CAVEATS AND PITFALLS
■ If prednisone is to be used for >21 days per course of therapy, obtain baseline chest radiograph, TB skin test & bone mineral density determination.
■ Check CBC Q2–3 weeks for 10–12 weeks w/ dapsone to detect rare pancytopenia.
■ Obtain baseline thiopurine methyltransferase level before starting azathioprine.
■ Closely monitor renal function & blood pressure w/ cyclosporine therapy.

DERMATOSIS PAPULOSA NIGRA

ALTERNATE DISEASE NAME
■ None

HISTORY
■ Hereditary predisposition
■ Occurs most frequently in black pts
■ Onset around time of puberty; new lesions throughout life

PHYSICAL EXAMINATION
- Multiple, firm, smooth, dark-brown to black, flattened papules
- Occur mainly on malar area of face & forehead

DIFFERENTIAL DIAGNOSIS
- Seborrheic keratosis
- Wart
- Nevocellular nevus
- Acrochordon (skin tag)
- Adenoma sebaceum

LABORATORY WORK-UP
- None

MANAGEMENT
- Destructive modality only for cosmetic reasons

SPECIFIC THERAPY
- Light electrodesiccation & curettage
- Cryotherapy

CAVEATS AND PITFALLS
- Advise about possible post-procedure dyspigmentation.

DERMOGRAPHISM

ALTERNATE DISEASE NAME
- Dermatographism
- Factitious urticaria
- Skin writing

HISTORY
- Occurs most commonly in young adults
- Pruritus may precede skin signs

PHYSICAL EXAMINATION
- Urticarial wheals develop within 5 minutes of stroking the skin
- Lesions persist for 15–30 minutes & resolve completely

DIFFERENTIAL DIAGNOSIS
- Chronic urticaria
- Contact urticaria

- Mastocytosis
- Insect bite reaction

LABORATORY WORK-UP
- Firm stroke of skin to produce linear wheal (Darier's sign)

MANAGEMENT
- Systemic antihistamines used chronically

SPECIFIC THERAPY
- Cetirizine 10 mg PO QD
- Fexofenadine 180 mg PO QD
- Loratadine 10 mg PO QD
- Desloratadine 5 mg PO QD

CAVEATS AND PITFALLS
- Eruption may persist for months or longer, requiring antihistamine suppression for that length of time.

DERMOID CYST

ALTERNATE DISEASE NAME
- Dermoid
- Choristoma
- Lipodermoid

HISTORY
- Occurs in infants

PHYSICAL EXAMINATION
- Appears most commonly on head & neck, particularly over supraorbital region, glabella, upper eyelid & scalp
- Subcutaneous mass, often w/ a dimple or sinus tract
- May contain nails, dental structures, cartilage-like & bone-like material & fat
- Deeper extension may cause lesion to be bound to underlying periosteum

DIFFERENTIAL DIAGNOSIS
- Epidermoid cyst
- Lymph node
- Pilomatricoma

- Thyroglossal duct cyst
- Meningocele or encephalocele
- Nevus sebaceus
- Cutaneous ectopic brain
- Metastasis

LABORATORY WORK-UP
- Imaging studies if there is a question of CNS connection

MANAGEMENT
- Surgical excision

SPECIFIC THERAPY
- Elliptical excision

CAVEATS AND PITFALLS
- CNS abnormalities possible if there is a direct connection.

DIGITAL MUCOUS CYST

ALTERNATE DISEASE NAME
- Mucous cyst
- Myxoid cyst
- Synovial cyst
- Digital mucoid cyst
- Digital myxoid cyst
- Myxomatous cyst
- Myxomatous degenerative cyst
- Digital mucinous pseudocyst

HISTORY
- May occur in context of distal digital osteoarthritis
- Asymptomatic unless traumatized

PHYSICAL EXAMINATION
- Solitary, round to oval, dome-shaped papule w/ normal overlying skin
- Contains a viscous, gelatinous, clear or yellow-tinged fluid

DIFFERENTIAL DIAGNOSIS
- Epidermoid cyst

- Fibrokeratoma
- Giant-cell tendon sheath tumor
- Heberden node
- Rheumatoid nodule
- Gouty tophus
- Subcutaneous granuloma annulare
- Myxoid malignant fibrous histiocytoma
- Myxoid variant of liposarcoma

LABORATORY WORK-UP
- None

MANAGEMENT
- Destructive modalities
- Incision & drainage
- Intralesional corticosteroids

SPECIFIC THERAPY
- Destruction by cryotherapy or electrodesiccation
- Surgical excision
- Intralesional triamcinolone 3–5 mg/mL

CAVEATS AND PITFALLS
- Frequent recurrences if lesion is not completely removed.

DILATED PORE

ALTERNATE DISEASE NAME
- Dilated pore of Winer
- Winer's pore
- Winer's dilated pore
- Giant hair follicle
- Enlarged solitary comedo

HISTORY
- Occurs in adults

PHYSICAL EXAMINATION
- Solitary large comedo, most commonly on back but also on face
- Lateral pressure produces keratinous material

DIFFERENTIAL DIAGNOSIS
- Epidermoid cyst
- Solar comedo
- Trichoepithelioma
- Pilar sheath acanthoma
- Trichofolliculoma

LABORATORY WORK-UP
- None

MANAGEMENT
- Destruction, only for cosmetic reasons

SPECIFIC THERAPY
- Expression of comedo contents, followed by electrodesiccation of base

CAVEATS AND PITFALLS
- Frequent recurrence if lesion is not completely destroyed.

DISSECTING CELLULITIS OF SCALP

ALTERNATE DISEASE NAME
- Dissecting cellulitis
- Perifolliculitis capitis abscedens et suffodiens
- Hoffman's disease

HISTORY
- Affects primarily black men
- May occur in association w/ acne conglobata & hidradenitis suppurativa (follicular occlusion triad)

PHYSICAL EXAMINATION
- Perifollicular pustules
- Tender nodules, some that discharge pus or gelatinous material
- Intercommunicating sinuses between nodules
- Patchy alopecia w/ scarring
- Frequent recurrences over many years

DIFFERENTIAL DIAGNOSIS
- Folliculitis keloidalis

- Folliculitis decalvans
- Bacterial pyoderma
- Kerion
- Pseudopelade of Brocq
- Lichen planopilaris

LABORATORY WORK-UP
- Bacterial & fungal culture
- Scalp biopsy if diagnosis is in doubt

MANAGEMENT
- Systemic anti-inflammatory agents
- Intralesional corticosteroid injection
- Laser hair removal
- Surgical incision or excision
  - ➤ Intralesional triamcinolone 3–5 mg/mL
  - ➤ Laser hair removal
  - ➤ Incision & drainage of fluctuant nodules
  - ➤ Wide local excision

SPECIFIC THERAPY
- Isotretinoin 1 mg/kg per day for 4–6 months
- Dapsone 50–200 mg PO QD indefinitely

CAVEATS AND PITFALLS
- Advise about the absolute contraindication of pregnancy during isotretinoin use.
- Check CBC Q 2–3 weeks for the first 10–12 weeks to detect rare pancytopenia with dapsone.
  - ➤ Obtain baseline G6PD level before dapsone therapy.

DYSHIDROTIC ECZEMA

ALTERNATE DISEASE NAME
- Dyshidrosis
- Pompholyx
- Vesicular palmoplantar eczema
- Vesicular eczema of palms & soles

HISTORY
- May be associated w/ atopy & emotional stress
- Chronic recurrent episodes over many years

PHYSICAL EXAMINATION
- Symmetrical crops of clear vesicles and/or bullae on palms & lateral aspects of fingers & feet
- Deep-seated vesicles, w/ a tapioca-like appearance
- Vesicles may become confluent to form bullae
- Crusting, scaling & fissuring after persistent scratching

DIFFERENTIAL DIAGNOSIS
- Contact dermatitis
- Vesicular tinea pedis
- Tinea manum
- Palmoplantar pustular psoriasis
- Autosensitization reaction (id reaction)

LABORATORY WORK-UP
- Potassium hydroxide preparation to rule out tinea pedis
- Bacterial culture if lesions are purulent

MANAGEMENT
- Topical corticosteroids
- Systemic corticosteroids
- Corticosteroid-sparing agents

SPECIFIC THERAPY
- Mild to moderate flare
  - Fluocinonide 0.05% cream applied BID
- Severe flare
  - Prednisone 1 mg/kg PO QD for 7–14 days
  - Triamcinolone 40–80 mg IM as single dose
- Chronic persistent disease
  - Corticosteroid-sparing agents
    - Azathioprine 2–3 mg/kg PO QD
    - Methotrexate 5–7.5 mg PO Q7 days
    - Cyclosporine 3–5 mg/kg PO QD
    - Local photochemotherapy (PUVA)

CAVEATS AND PITFALLS

■ Use prednisone for no longer than 21 days per treatment course unless there is very severe disease.

■ If prednisone is to be used for >21 days per course of therapy, obtain baseline chest radiograph, TB skin test & bone mineral density determination.

■ Check CBC Q2–3 weeks for 10–12 weeks w/ dapsone to detect rare pancytopenia.

■ Obtain baseline thiopurine methyltransferase level before starting azathioprine.

■ Closely monitor renal function & blood pressure w/ cyclosporine therapy.

DYSKERATOSIS CONGENITA

ALTERNATE DISEASE NAME

■ Zinsser-Engman-Cole syndrome

■ Zinsser-Cole-Engman syndrome

HISTORY

■ 90% in males w/ familial clustering

■ Bone marrow dysfunction & subsequent failure

■ Predisposition to malignancies, including mucosal squamous cell carcinoma, Hodgkin's disease & leukemia

PHYSICAL EXAMINATION

■ Skin manifestations begin between 5 & 15 years of age

■ Tan to gray, hyperpigmented or hypopigmented macules & patches in a mottled or reticulated pattern, sometimes w/ poikiloderma

■ Skin changes on upper trunk, neck & face, often w/ involvement of sun-exposed areas

■ Progressive nail dystrophy & scalp alopecia

■ Leukokeratosis on buccal mucosa, tongue, oropharynx, esophagus, urethral meatus, glans penis, lacrimal duct, conjunctiva, vagina & anus

■ Dental caries

DIFFERENTIAL DIAGNOSIS
- Graft-versus-host disease
- Fanconi syndrome
- Rothmund-Thompson syndrome
- Ataxia-telangiectasia

LABORATORY WORK-UP
- None

MANAGEMENT
- Sun & cigarette avoidance
- Bone marrow transplantation

SPECIFIC THERAPY
- See "Management"

CAVEATS AND PITFALLS
- None

ECCRINE ACROSPIROMA

ALTERNATE DISEASE NAME
- Acrospiroma
- Myoepithelioma
- Clear cell hidradenoma
- Clear cell adenoma
- Cystic hidradenoma
- Sweat gland adenoma
- Eccrine sweat gland adenoma

HISTORY
- Presents as slow-growing lesion in adults
- May appear after minor trauma

PHYSICAL EXAMINATION
- Solitary, flesh-colored dermal papule; occurs most commonly on scalp, face & trunk, w/ tendency for central ulceration
- Occasional malignant degeneration

DIFFERENTIAL DIAGNOSIS
- Basal cell carcinoma

- Lymphangioma
- Hemangioma
- Squamous cell carcinoma

LABORATORY WORK-UP
- Lesional biopsy for routine histology

MANAGEMENT
- Surgical excision

SPECIFIC THERAPY
- See "Management"

CAVEATS AND PITFALLS
- None

ECCRINE SPIRADENOMA

ALTERNATE DISEASE NAME
- Spiradenoma

HISTORY
- Appears as slow-growing lesion in adults

PHYSICAL EXAMINATION
- Solitary firm, gray-pink papule, usually arising in head & neck region or trunk
- Occasional pain & tenderness

DIFFERENTIAL DIAGNOSIS
- Cylindroma
- Basal cell carcinoma
- Trichoepithelioma
- Eccrine poroma
- Angiofibroma
- Milium

LABORATORY WORK-UP
- Lesional biopsy for routine histology

MANAGEMENT
- Surgical excision

SPECIFIC THERAPY
- See "Management"

CAVEATS AND PITFALLS
- None

ECTHYMA GANGRENOSUM

ALTERNATE DISEASE NAME
- None

HISTORY
- Occurs in immunocompromised or otherwise debilitated pts
- Manifestation of widespread *Pseudomonas* sepsis

PHYSICAL EXAMINATION
- Presents as edematous, well-circumscribed plaques, rapidly evolving into hemorrhagic bullae
- Spreads peripherally & eventually develops a black necrotic ulcer w/ an erythematous rim, often on gluteal or perineal region or extremities

DIFFERENTIAL DIAGNOSIS
- Septicemia from other infectious agents
- Ecthyma
- Necrotizing fasciitis
- Herpes simplex virus infection
- Atypical tuberculosis
- Nocardiosis
- Sporotrichosis
- Gram-negative folliculitis
- Pyoderma gangrenosum
- Trauma
- Cryoglobulinemia
- Polyarteritis nodosa

LABORATORY WORK-UP
- Wound culture for bacterial pathogens
- Blood cultures

MANAGEMENT
- Systemic antibiotics

SPECIFIC THERAPY
- Initial therapy: antipseudomonal penicillin (piperacillin) w/ an aminoglycoside (gentamicin)
- Subsequent therapy based on culture & sensitivity

CAVEATS AND PITFALLS
- Life-threatening emergency.

ECZEMA HERPETICUM

ALTERNATE DISEASE NAME
- Kaposi varicelliform eruption
- Eczema vaccinatum

HISTORY
- Occurs in pts w/ active eczema & herpes virus colonization
- May also appear in the skin of those w/ other dermatoses such as pemphigus, Darier disease, burns & ichthyosis

PHYSICAL EXAMINATION
- Presents as clusters of umbilicated vesiculopustules in areas where the skin has been affected by a preexistent dermatitis, usually over upper trunk & head
- Umbilicated vesicles and/or pustules that progress to erosions
- May become hemorrhagic & crusted & coalesce to form eroded plaques
- May develop secondary bacterial infection

DIFFERENTIAL DIAGNOSIS
- Impetigo
- Varicella
- Erythema multiforme
- Contact dermatitis
- Bullous pemphigoid
- Dermatitis herpetiformis
- Pemphigus vulgaris

LABORATORY WORK-UP
- Lesion culture for herpes virus

MANAGEMENT
- Systemic antiviral agents

SPECIFIC THERAPY
- Acyclovir
  - Adult dosage: 500 mg IV/day divided into 3 doses for 5 days
  - Pediatric dosage: 15 mg/kg IV per day divided into 3 doses for 5 days
- Valacyclovir
  - Adult dosage: 1,000 mg PO BID for 10 days
  - Pediatric dosage: not established

CAVEATS AND PITFALLS
- Herpes virus culture positive only when taken from intact vesicle.

EHLERS-DANLOS SYNDROME

ALTERNATE DISEASE NAME
- Cutis hyperelastica

HISTORY
- Heritable group of diseases w/ common findings of connective tissue pathology
- Skin changes noted at birth in many cases

PHYSICAL EXAMINATION
- Hyperextensible, doughy, white & soft skin, w/ underlying vessels often visible
- Small, spongy tumors (molluscoid pseudotumors) over scars & pressure points
- Deep, palpable & movable calcified papules in subcutaneous tissue
- Skin fragility, w/ frequent bruises, lacerations & poor wound healing
- Hyperextensible joints, w/ frequent dislocations

DIFFERENTIAL DIAGNOSIS
- Pseudoxanthoma elasticum

- Marfan syndrome
- Cartilage-hair syndrome
- Cutis laxa
- Turner's syndrome

LABORATORY WORK-UP
- None

MANAGEMENT
- Avoid contact sports
- Genetic counseling

SPECIFIC THERAPY
- None

CAVEATS AND PITFALLS
- Avoid surgery, if possible, because of poor wound healing.

ELASTOSIS PERFORANS SERPIGINOSA

ALTERNATE DISEASE NAME
- Elastosis perforans serpiginosum
- Reactive perforating elastosis
- Elastosis perforans
- Elastosis intrapapillare
- Elastoma intrapapillare perforans
- Elastoma verruciform perforans
- Keratosis follicularis serpiginosa

HISTORY
- Onset in childhood or early adulthood
- Associated w/ Down's syndrome, Ehlers-Danlos syndrome, Marfan syndrome, osteogenesis imperfecta, scleroderma, acrogeria, pseudoxanthoma elasticum & w/ penicillamine use

PHYSICAL EXAMINATION
- Flesh-colored or pale-red, umbilicated papules grouped in linear, arciform, circular or serpiginous patterns
- Occurs most commonly over nape of neck

DIFFERENTIAL DIAGNOSIS
- Reactive perforating collagenosis
- Perforating folliculitis
- Kyrle's disease
- Folliculitis
- Prurigo nodularis
- Granuloma annulare
- Tinea corporis
- Lupus erythematosus

LABORATORY WORK-UP
- Skin biopsy if diagnosis is in doubt

MANAGEMENT
- Systemic or topical retinoids
- Destructive surgical modalities

SPECIFIC THERAPY
- Retinoids
  - Tretinoin 0.025% cream applied QD for months
  - Isotretinoin 0.5 mg/kg PO QD for 1 month followed by 1 mg/kg per day for 4 months
- Destructive modalities
  - Cryotherapy
  - Electrodesiccation & curettage

CAVEATS AND PITFALLS
- Commonly recurs if not excised completely.
- Absolute contraindication of isotretinoin in pregnancy.

EOSINOPHILIC CELLULITIS

ALTERNATE DISEASE NAME
- Wells' syndrome
- Wells syndrome
- Recurrent granulomatous dermatitis w/ eosinophilia

HISTORY
- Recurrent episodes of pruritus & an eruption, lasting 4–8 weeks
- Occasional malaise & fever

PHYSICAL EXAMINATION
- Pruritus & burning sensation, followed by cellulitis-like eruption
- Large, indurated plaques of edema & erythema, w/ violaceous borders
- May also have annular plaques, papules & urticarial wheals

DIFFERENTIAL DIAGNOSIS
- Cellulitis
- Erysipelas
- Urticaria
- Hypereosinophilic syndrome
- Insect bite reaction
- Lyme disease
- Inflammatory metastasis
- Granuloma annulare
- Churg-Strauss syndrome

LABORATORY WORK-UP
- Skin biopsy
- CBC, looking for peripheral eosinophilia

MANAGEMENT
- Systemic corticosteroids

SPECIFIC THERAPY
- Prednisone 1 mg/kg PO QD for 2–4 weeks

CAVEATS AND PITFALLS
- Taper prednisone over 2–6 weeks if at full dose at 21 days.
- Some association w/ myeloproliferative disorders

EOSINOPHILIC PUSTULAR FOLLICULITIS

ALTERNATE DISEASE NAME
- Ofuji's disease
- Ofuji disease
- Eosinophilic folliculitis
- Infantile/childhood eosinophilic pustulosis of the scalp
- HIV-associated eosinophilic folliculitis
- HIV-related eosinophilic folliculitis

- Sterile eosinophilic pustulosis
- Eosinophilic pustular dermatosis

HISTORY
- Usual onset in neonatal period
- Complication of HIV disease

PHYSICAL EXAMINATION
- Follicular-based erythematous papules & pustules, which may coalesce into plaques
- Most commonly occurs on scalp in infants & on face, back & extensor surfaces of upper extremities in adults
- May have peripheral eosinophilia

DIFFERENTIAL DIAGNOSIS
- Other forms of folliculitis, including bacterial & fungal varieties
- Pustular psoriasis
- Acne vulgaris
- Rosacea
- Perioral dermatitis
- Scabies
- Insect bite reaction
- Langerhans cell histiocytosis
- Follicular mucinosis
- Pemphigus foliaceus

LABORATORY WORK-UP
- Skin biopsy for confirmation of diagnosis
- Gram stain of pustular contents
- Bacterial, fungal culture of intact pustule

MANAGEMENT
- May be self-limited, particularly in infants
- Sulfones
- Topical corticosteroids
- Systemic corticosteroids
- Phototherapy

SPECIFIC THERAPY
- Dapsone 25–100 mg PO QD

- Clobetasol 0.05% cream applied BID
- Prednisone 1 mg/kg PO QD for up to 3 weeks

CAVEATS AND PITFALLS
- With dapsone therapy, check CBC every 2–3 weeks for 10–12 weeks.
  - ➤ Obtain baseline G6PD level before dapsone therapy.
  - ➤ Some association w/ myeloproliferative disorders

EPHELIDES

ALTERNATE DISEASE NAME
- Freckles

HISTORY
- Occur on a familial basis, mainly in those w/ red or blond hair
- Appear within the first 2–3 years of life

PHYSICAL EXAMINATION
- Multiple, small, uniformly tan macules on sun-exposed skin, sometimes coalescing into patches
- Darken w/ sun exposure & lighten after prolonged sun avoidance

DIFFERENTIAL DIAGNOSIS
- Lentigo
- Seborrheic keratosis
- Melanocytic nevus
- Tinea versicolor
- Café-au-lait spot

LABORATORY WORK-UP
- None

MANAGEMENT
- Sun avoidance
- Sunscreens

SPECIFIC THERAPY
- None

CAVEATS AND PITFALLS
- None

EPIDERMODYSPLASIA VERRUCIFORMIS

ALTERNATE DISEASE NAME
- None

HISTORY
- Familial incidence
- Begins in childhood

PHYSICAL EXAMINATION
- Polymorphic, verrucous or flat-topped papules resembling flat warts
- Macules & reddish-brown plaques w/ slightly scaly surfaces & irregular borders
- Lesions are localized mostly on sun-exposed regions, palms, soles, in the axillae & on external genitalia
- Mucous membranes rarely affected
- Malignant tumors may appear during the fourth & fifth decades of life

DIFFERENTIAL DIAGNOSIS
- Verruca plana
- Squamous cell carcinoma
- Trichoepithelioma
- Basal cell carcinoma
- Papular mucinosis
- Solar elastosis
- Tinea versicolor

LABORATORY WORK-UP
- Lesional biopsy

MANAGEMENT
- Sun protection
- Destructive modalities for individual lesions

SPECIFIC THERAPY
- Cryotherapy
- Destruction by electrodesiccation & curettage

CAVEATS AND PITFALLS
- None

EPIDERMOID CYST

ALTERNATE DISEASE NAME
- Epidermal cyst
- Epidermal inclusion cyst
- Sebaceous cyst
- Wen
- Atheroma
- Steatoma

HISTORY
- Asymptomatic, slowly enlarging lesion
- May have history of multiple similar tumors

PHYSICAL EXAMINATION
- White or pale-yellow, deep dermal or subcutaneous, medium-firm papule or nodule, often w/ a central pore
- Cheesy, foul-smelling material may exude w/ lateral pressure

DIFFERENTIAL DIAGNOSIS
- Lipoma
- Cylindroma
- Trichilemmoma
- Steatocystoma multiplex
- Granuloma annulare
- Sarcoidosis
- Lymphocytic infiltration
- Insect bite reaction
- Acquired perforating disease
- Metastasis

LABORATORY WORK-UP
- None

MANAGEMENT
- Surgical excision only for cosmetic purposes or if lesion is symptomatic
  - Simple excision by sharp dissection
  - Elliptical excision
    - Marsupialization of large nodules
- Intralesional corticosteroids for inflamed lesion

SPECIFIC THERAPY

■ Inflamed lesion

➤ Incision & drainage of purulent material

➤ Triamcinolone (3–5 mg/mL) injected intralesionally

CAVEATS AND PITFALLS

■ Frequent recurrences if lesion not completely excised or if cyst sac is not completely removed.

EPIDERMOLYSIS BULLOSA

ALTERNATE DISEASE NAME

■ None

HISTORY

■ Skin fragility & blistering at sites of minor trauma

■ May begin at birth or later in life, depending on the type

PHYSICAL EXAMINATION

■ Epidermolysis bullosa simplex

➤ Weber-Cockayne type

• Most common form

• Usually appears on palms & soles, often w/ hyperhidrosis

➤ Dowling-Meara type: involves oral mucosa w/ grouped herpetiform blisters

➤ Koebner type: palmoplantar hyperkeratosis & erosions

➤ Severe type

• Generalized onset of blisters occurring at or shortly after birth

• Hands, feet & extremities most common sites of involvement

■ Junctional epidermolysis bullosa

➤ Letalis (Herlitz) type

• Generalized blistering at birth, w/ poor prognosis

• Orificial erosions around mouth, eyes & nares, often w/ excess granulation tissue

• Involvement of corneal, conjunctival, tracheobronchial, oral, pharyngeal, esophageal, rectal & genitourinary mucosal surfaces

- Internal complications include hoarse cry, cough & other respiratory difficulties
  - ➤ Nonlethal junctional type (mitis form)
    - Generalized blistering, which improves w/ age
    - Scalp, nail & tooth abnormalities
    - Periorificial erosions & hypertrophic granulation tissue
    - Mucous membrane erosions, resulting in strictures
- ■ Dystrophic epidermolysis bullosa
  - ➤ Dominantly inherited type
    - Onset of disease usually at birth or during infancy, w/ generalized blistering
    - Evolution to localized blistering w/ age
- ■ Cockayne-Touraine type
  - ➤ Acral distribution
  - ➤ Minimal oral involvement
- ■ Pasini type
  - ➤ More extensive blistering w/ scarlike papules on trunk (albopapuloid lesions)
  - ➤ Oral mucosa & teeth involvement
  - ➤ Dystrophic or absent nails
- ■ Mitis type
  - ➤ Involves acral areas & nails
  - ➤ Usually spares mucosal surfaces
  - ➤ Clinical manifestations similar to dominantly inherited forms
- ■ Severe recessive variant (Hallopeau-Siemens)
  - ➤ Generalized blistering at birth, w/ subsequent extensive dystrophic scarring
  - ➤ Most prominent on acral surfaces, sometimes resulting in pseudosyndactyly (mitten-hand deformity) of hands & feet
  - ➤ Flexion contractures of extremities w/ age
  - ➤ Dystrophy of nails & teeth
  - ➤ Involvement of internal mucosa, sometimes causing esophageal strictures & webs
  - ➤ Urethral & anal stenosis, phimosis & corneal scarring
  - ➤ Intestinal malabsorption leading to a mixed anemia resulting from lack of iron absorption & failure to thrive
  - ➤ Risk of developing squamous cell carcinomas in areas of chronic blistering

DIFFERENTIAL DIAGNOSIS
- Friction blisters
- Linear IgA bullous disease
- Bullous pemphigoid
- Epidermolysis bullosa acquisita
- Pemphigus vulgaris
- Thermal or chemical burn

LABORATORY WORK-UP
- None

MANAGEMENT
- Avoidance of frictional trauma
- Careful attention to skin & dental hygiene

SPECIFIC THERAPY
- Severe disease
  - ➤ Soft diet to prevent esophageal trauma & blistering
  - ➤ Skin-equivalent dressings & grafts to promote epithelialization

CAVEATS AND PITFALLS
- Malnutrition is potential complication of severe oral involvement.

EPIDERMOLYSIS BULLOSA ACQUISITA

ALTERNATE DISEASE NAME
- Acquired epidermolysis bullosa
- EBA

HISTORY
- Gradual onset of skin fragility in trauma-prone skin
- Subset w/ abrupt onset of generalized blistering, not only in trauma-prone skin
- Affects mainly elderly individuals

PHYSICAL EXAMINATION
- Noninflammatory variant
  - ➤ Tense vesicles, bullae & erosions, primarily on extensor surfaces of hands, knuckles, elbows, knees & ankles

- Mucous membrane erosions
- Scarring & milia in affected areas
- Generalized inflammatory variant
  - Widespread distribution of tense vesicles & bullae
  - Generalized erythema, urticarial plaques & pruritus in some pts

DIFFERENTIAL DIAGNOSIS
- Bullous pemphigoid
- Porphyria cutanea tarda
- Epidermolysis bullosa
- Linear IgA bullous dermatosis
- Cicatricial pemphigoid

LABORATORY WORK-UP
- Skin biopsy for routine light microscopy
- Skin biopsy for direct immunofluorescence
- Serum for indirect immunofluorescence

MANAGEMENT
- Systemic corticosteroids
- Corticosteroid-sparing agents

SPECIFIC THERAPY
- Prednisone 1 mg/kg per day PO as a single AM dose
- Corticosteroid-sparing agents
  - Azathioprine 2–3 mg/kg per day
  - Dapsone 100–200 mg PO per day
  - Colchicine 0.6–1.8 mg PO per day
  - Cyclosporine 3–5 mg/kg PO per day

CAVEATS AND PITFALLS
- Before starting chronic prednisone therapy, obtain TB skin test, chest radiograph & bone density scan & vitamin D & calcium supplementation.
- Check CBC Q2–3 weeks for 10–12 weeks w/ dapsone to detect rare pancytopenia.
- Obtain baseline thiopurine methyltransferase level before starting azathioprine.
- Closely monitor renal function & blood pressure w/ cyclosporine therapy.

ERYSIPELAS

ALTERNATE DISEASE NAME
- None

HISTORY
- Acute onset of fever, chills, myalgias, arthralgias & headache

PHYSICAL EXAMINATION
- Begins as small erythematous patch & evolves to red, indurated, shiny plaque
- Raised, sharply demarcated plaque, w/ advancing margins, skin warmth, edema & tenderness
- Lymphatic involvement w/ overlying skin streaking & regional lymphadenopathy

DIFFERENTIAL DIAGNOSIS
- Contact dermatitis
- Seborrheic dermatitis
- Lupus erythematosus
- Angioedema
- Herpes zoster
- Erysipeloid
- Necrotizing fasciitis

LABORATORY WORK-UP
- Blood cultures

MANAGEMENT
- Systemic antibiotics

SPECIFIC THERAPY
- Streptococcal infection
  - 1.2 million units as a single IM injection
  - Cephalexin 250–500 mg PO QID for 7 days; use if pt is allergic to penicillin
- Staphylococcal infection
  - Penicillin G procaine 1.2 million units as a single IM injection

➤ Dicloxacillin 500 mg PO QID for 10 days
➤ Cephalexin 250–500 mg PO QID for 7 days; use if pt is allergic to penicillin

CAVEATS AND PITFALLS
■ Recurrences common if there is lymphatic sclerosis at drainage site.

ERYSIPELOID

ALTERNATE DISEASE NAME
■ Erysipeloid of Rosenbach

HISTORY
■ Occurs mainly in food handlers, such as butchers, fishermen & homemakers
■ Presents w/ local burning or pain at lesion sites, w/ or w/o fever, malaise & other constitutional symptoms

PHYSICAL EXAMINATION
■ Localized form
   ➤ Well-demarcated, bright-red to purple, warm, tender plaques w/ a smooth, shiny surface
   ➤ Occurs most commonly on hands
■ Diffuse cutaneous form
   ➤ Multiple, well-demarcated, violaceous plaques w/ an advancing border & central clearing
■ Systemic form
   ➤ Localized areas of swelling surrounding a necrotic center
   ➤ May present as follicular, erythematous papules
   ➤ Endocarditis & septicemia are potential complications

DIFFERENTIAL DIAGNOSIS
■ Cellulitis
■ Erysipelas
■ Fixed drug reaction
■ Erythema nodosum
■ Leishmaniasis

LABORATORY WORK-UP
- Gram stain & bacterial culture
- Blood cultures for suspected systemic erysipeloid
- Skin biopsy to confirm diagnosis

MANAGEMENT
- Systemic antibiotics

SPECIFIC THERAPY
- Penicillin VK 250–500 mg PO QID for 10 days
- Erythromycin 250–500 mg PO QID & rifampin 600 mg PO QD for 7–10 days in penicillin-allergic pts

CAVEATS AND PITFALLS
- None

ERYTHEMA AB IGNE

ALTERNATE DISEASE NAME
- Erythema ab igne elastosis
- Toasted skin syndrome
- Ephelis ab igne
- Erythema à calore

HISTORY
- Short-term or long-term localized excess heat exposure from radiant sources such as fireplaces, heating pads or hot water bottles

PHYSICAL EXAMINATION
- Reticulated violaceous & hyperpigmented plaques, most common on the legs of women
- Poikiloderma w/ severe long-standing disease

DIFFERENTIAL DIAGNOSIS
- Livedo reticularis
- Poikiloderma of Civatte
- Poikiloderma atrophicans vasculare
- Morphea
- Livedo vasculitis

LABORATORY WORK-UP
- Skin biopsy, only if there is doubt about the diagnosis

MANAGEMENT
- Avoid localized hyperthermia
- Laser ablation using Nd:YAG, ruby or alexandrite laser

SPECIFIC THERAPY
- See "Management"

CAVEATS AND PITFALLS
- Cumulative skin damage w/ repeat heat exposures.
- Incomplete response to laser therapy.

ERYTHEMA ANNULARE CENTRIFUGUM

ALTERNATE DISEASE NAME
- Erythema gyratum perstans
- Erythema perstans
- Erythema exudativum perstans
- Erythema marginatum perstans
- Erythema figuratum perstans
- Erythema simplex gyratum

HISTORY
- May have preceding infection or new use of medication
- May have associated underlying disease, such as malignancy or other systemic illness w/ characteristic symptoms (eg, night sweats, fever)

PHYSICAL EXAMINATION
- Starts as asymptomatic, erythematous papules & spreads peripherally while clearing centrally, often w/ a trailing scale on the inner aspect of the advancing edge
- Appears on any skin surface other than palms & soles

DIFFERENTIAL DIAGNOSIS
- Tinea corporis
- Erythema marginatum
- Erythema migrans
- Granuloma annulare

- Sarcoidosis
- Urticaria
- Erythema gyratum repens
- Seborrheic dermatitis
- Lupus erythematosus
- Benign lymphocytic infiltrate

LABORATORY WORK-UP
- KOH examination of skin scraping to rule out dermatophyte infection

MANAGEMENT
- Discontinue suspect medications
- Internal medicine work-up directed to localizing signs & symptoms
- Topical corticosteroids
- Systemic corticosteroids only for very symptomatic pts; limit therapy to <3 weeks

SPECIFIC THERAPY
- Clobetasol 0.05% cream applied BID
- Prednisone 1 mg/kg PO QD for up to 3 weeks

CAVEATS AND PITFALLS
- Limited benefit of topical or systemic corticosteroid therapy; does not shorten course of disease.

ERYTHEMA ELEVATUM DIUTINUM

ALTERNATE DISEASE NAME
- Extracellular cholesterosis
- EED

HISTORY
- Occasional history of arthralgia
- Sudden onset of asymptomatic lesions

PHYSICAL EXAMINATION
- Red to violaceous, smooth, brown or yellow papules, plaques or nodules over extensor surfaces, especially over joints
- Occasional vesiculation, crusting or bleeding

DIFFERENTIAL DIAGNOSIS
- Granuloma annulare
- Sarcoidosis
- Insect bite reaction
- Rheumatoid nodules
- Gouty tophi
- Xanthomas
- Multicentric reticulohistiocytosis
- Erythema multiforme
- Acute neutrophilic dermatosis

LABORATORY WORK-UP
- Skin biopsy

MANAGEMENT
- Sulfones

SPECIFIC THERAPY
- Dapsone 100 mg PO QD; titrate as per response

CAVEATS AND PITFALLS
- Check CBC Q2–3 weeks for 10–12 weeks w/ dapsone to detect rare pancytopenia.
  - Obtain baseline G6PD level before dapsone therapy.

ERYTHEMA MULTIFORME

ALTERNATE DISEASE NAME
- Erythema exudativum
- Hebra's disease
- Erythema polymorphe

HISTORY
- Preceding infection (often HSV infection or streptococcal infection) or medication ingestion
- Occasionally associated w/ rheumatic diseases, vasculitides, non-Hodgkin lymphoma, leukemia, multiple myeloma, myeloid metaplasia or polycythemia vera
- With EM major, may have prodrome of moderate fever, general discomfort, cough, sore throat, vomiting, chest pain & diarrhea

PHYSICAL EXAMINATION
- Erythema multiforme minor variant
  - Initial lesion is dull-red macule or urticarial plaque, sometimes w/ small papule, vesicle or bulla centrally
  - Raised, pale, edematous ring at the periphery, gradually becoming violaceous & forming concentric target lesion
  - Lesions are located predominantly on the extensor surfaces of acral extremities & spread centripetally
  - Mild erosions of one mucosal surface
  - Palms, neck & face frequently involved
- Erythema multiforme major variant
  - Skin lesions same as w/ erythema multiforme minor
  - Severe erosions of at least 2 mucosal surfaces
  - Generalized lymphadenopathy

DIFFERENTIAL DIAGNOSIS
- Urticaria
- Figurate erythema
- Stevens-Johnson syndrome
- Toxic epidermal necrolysis
- Henoch-Schönlein purpura
- Viral exanthem
- Kawasaki disease
- Fixed drug eruption
- Lupus erythematosus
- Primary herpetic gingivostomatitis
- Aphthous stomatitis
- Behçet disease
- Bullous pemphigoid

LABORATORY WORK-UP
- EM major work-up
  - CBC
  - Electrolyte levels
  - BUN determination
  - Erythrocyte sedimentation rate (ESR)
  - Liver function tests
  - Cultures from blood, sputum & erosive areas

MANAGEMENT
- Systemic antihistamines
- Systemic corticosteroids
- Herpes simplex virus prophylaxis for recurrent episodes (>4 or 5 episodes per year)

SPECIFIC THERAPY
- Doxepin 10–50 mg PO QHS
- Prednisone 1 mg/kg PO QAM for 7–14 days
- Herpes simplex virus prophylaxis: valacyclovir 500–1,000 mg PO QD for up to 1 year

CAVEATS AND PITFALLS
- Use prednisone only after ruling out systemic infection.

ERYTHEMA NODOSUM

ALTERNATE DISEASE NAME
- Dermatitis contusiformis
- Erythema contusiformis
- Focal septal panniculitis
- Nodose fever

HISTORY
- Prodrome of flu-like symptoms, w/ fever & generalized myalgia
- Often a preceding or concomitant infection such as strep, coccidioidomycosis or tuberculosis
- Occasional causative agent is oral contraceptives or sulfonamides

PHYSICAL EXAMINATION
- Lesions present as poorly defined, red, tender nodules, which become firm & painful during the 2d week
- Associated leg edema & pain
- Lesions may become fluctuant but do not suppurate or ulcerate
- Individual lesions last approximately 2 weeks

DIFFERENTIAL DIAGNOSIS
- Nodular vasculitis
- Erysipelas
- Cellulitis

- Superficial thrombophlebitis
- Weber-Christian disease
- Pancreatic panniculitis
- Lupus profundus
- Traumatic panniculitis
- Polyarteritis nodosa
- Insect bite reaction

LABORATORY WORK-UP
- Throat culture to rule out group A beta-hemolytic streptococcal infection
- Chest radiograph as part of the initial workup to exclude sarcoidosis, tuberculosis & coccidioidomycosis
- Deep skin incisional biopsy if diagnosis is in doubt

MANAGEMENT
- Nonsteroidal anti-inflammatory agents
- Bed rest
- Leg elevation
- Systemic corticosteroids

SPECIFIC THERAPY
- Prednisone 1 mg/kg PO QAM for a maximum of 21 days

CAVEATS AND PITFALLS
- Biopsy must include subcutaneous fat.
- Use prednisone only for short courses in severe, recalcitrant cases not responding to other measures.

ERYTHEMA TOXICUM

ALTERNATE DISEASE NAME
- Erythema toxicum neonatorum
- Erythema neonatorum
- Toxic erythema
- Erythema neonatorum allergicum
- Erythema papulosum
- Urticaria neonatorum
- Erythema dyspepsicum

HISTORY
- Usually occurs within first 4 days of life in full-term infants
- Infants are typically otherwise healthy

PHYSICAL EXAMINATION
- Presents as a patchy, evanescent, macular erythema, often on face or trunk
- Sites of predilection include forehead, face, trunk & proximal extremities, but may occur anywhere except for mucous membranes

DIFFERENTIAL DIAGNOSIS
- Urticaria
- Transient neonatal pustular melanosis
- Candidiasis
- Miliaria
- Pyoderma
- Varicella
- Herpes simplex virus infection
- Folliculitis
- Insect bite reaction

LABORATORY WORK-UP
- Gram stain of contents of vesicle, looking for sheets of eosinophils

MANAGEMENT
- None

SPECIFIC THERAPY
- None

CAVEATS AND PITFALLS
- None

ERYTHRASMA

ALTERNATE DISEASE NAME
- None

HISTORY
- Occurs most commonly in warm, moist environments

- Predisposing factors include excessive sweating & hyperhidrosis, disrupted cutaneous barrier, obesity, diabetes mellitus & immunocompromised states
- Caused by bacterial pathogen, *Corynebacterium minutissimum*

PHYSICAL EXAMINATION
- Well-demarcated, brown-red, minimally scaly plaques, often over inner thighs, crural region, scrotum & toe webs or other intertriginous sites
- Toe web lesions appear macerated

DIFFERENTIAL DIAGNOSIS
- Intertrigo
- Tinea pedis
- Tinea corporis
- Tinea cruris
- Contact dermatitis
- Dyshidrotic eczema
- Contact dermatitis

LABORATORY WORK-UP
- Wood's light exam, looking for coral red fluorescence

MANAGEMENT
- Topical anti-infective agents
- Systemic antibiotics
- Drying powders

SPECIFIC THERAPY
- Topical anti-infective agents
  - Miconazole cream applied BID for 3–4 weeks
  - Clotrimazole cream applied BID for 3–4 weeks
- Systemic antibiotics
  - Erythromycin base 500 mg PO QID for 7–10 days
  - Clarithromycin 1,000 mg PO for 1 dose

CAVEATS AND PITFALLS
- None

ERYTHROMELALGIA

ALTERNATE DISEASE NAME
- Erythermalgia

HISTORY
- Signs & symptoms brought on by warming or dependency & relieved by cooling
- No signs or symptoms between attacks
- Most cases unrelated to other illnesses
- Occasional association w/ myeloproliferative disorder or rheumatic disease

PHYSICAL EXAMINATION
- Red, painful, warm extremities brought on by warming or dependency, lasting minutes to days, relieved by cooling
- Lower extremities affected more often than upper extremities

DIFFERENTIAL DIAGNOSIS
- Raynaud phenomenon
- Reflex sympathetic dystrophy
- Cellulitis
- Vasculitis
- Frostbite

LABORATORY WORK-UP
- Platelet count

MANAGEMENT
- Cooling or elevating extremity to relieve symptoms of attack
- Aspirin

SPECIFIC THERAPY
- Aspirin 500 mg PO prn

CAVEATS AND PITFALLS
- Aspirin is useful only in pts w/ thrombocytosis.

ERYTHROPOIETIC PROTOPORPHYRIA

ALTERNATE DISEASE NAME
- Erythrohepatic protoporphyria
- Congenital erythropoietic protoporphyria
- Protoporphyria

HISTORY
- Usual onset in infancy or early childhood
- Acute attack after few minutes of sun exposure
- Acute reaction is painful & resolves over several days

PHYSICAL EXAMINATION
- Immediate edema, erythema & petechiae after sun exposure, w/ occasional vesiculation
- Chronic skin changes include facial scars, perioral furrowing & aged-appearing, thickened or hyperkeratotic skin of the dorsal hands
- After sustained, more intense or frequent sun exposure, waxy scleroderma-like induration and/or weather-beaten or cobblestone texture of the face & dorsal aspects of hands
- Rare progressive liver failure, w/ hepatosplenomegaly & jaundice

DIFFERENTIAL DIAGNOSIS
- Polymorphous light eruption
- Light-sensitive atopic dermatitis
- Solar urticaria
- Acute tar photosensitivity
- Hereditary coproporphyria
- Porphyria cutanea tarda
- Pseudoporphyria

LABORATORY WORK-UP
- Erythrocyte & plasma protoporphyrin levels
- CBC, liver function studies for baseline evaluation

MANAGEMENT
- Sun avoidance
- Carotenoids

SPECIFIC THERAPY
- Beta-carotene 120–300 mg PO per day

CAVEATS AND PITFALLS
- Carotenoids of only limited benefit.

FAMILIAL BENIGN CHRONIC PEMPHIGUS

ALTERNATE DISEASE NAME
- Hailey-Hailey disease
- Familial benign pemphigus

HISTORY
- Common familial pattern
- Symptoms & signs may not begin until after age 30 years
- Worsened w/ heat, friction & secondary infection

PHYSICAL EXAMINATION
- Vesicles & erythematous plaques w/ overlying crusts, often in the genital area, chest, neck & axillary areas
- Burning sensation & pruritus
- Malodorous drainage w/ secondary infection

DIFFERENTIAL DIAGNOSIS
- Darier disease
- Impetigo
- Candidiasis
- Atopic dermatitis
- Seborrheic dermatitis
- Herpes simplex virus infection
- Pemphigus vulgaris
- Pemphigus foliaceous
- Extramammary Paget's disease

LABORATORY WORK-UP
- Skin biopsy

MANAGEMENT
- Topical corticosteroids
- Topical antibiotics
- Systemic antibiotics
- Surgical ablation w/ laser ablation or dermabrasion

SPECIFIC THERAPY
- Triamcinolone 0.1% cream applied BID
- Clindamycin 1% solution applied BID
- Erythromycin 2% solution applied BID
- Erythromycin base 500 mg PO QID

CAVEATS AND PITFALLS
- Systemic antibiotics used only for secondary infection.

FAVRE-RACOUCHOT DISEASE

ALTERNATE DISEASE NAME
- Syndrome of Favre-Racouchot
- Senile comedones
- Solar comedones
- Nodular cutaneous elastoidosis w/ cysts & comedones
- Smoker's comedones

HISTORY
- Chronic sun exposure
- Cigarette smoking is major risk factor

PHYSICAL EXAMINATION
- Multiple, bilaterally symmetrical, open & closed comedos in periorbital & temporal areas
- Occasionally noted in lateral neck, postauricular areas & forearms
- Actinically damaged skin w/ yellowish discoloration, yellowish nodules, atrophy, wrinkles & furrows

DIFFERENTIAL DIAGNOSIS
- Sebaceous hyperplasia
- Acne vulgaris
- Nevus comedonicus
- Colloid milia
- Milia
- Trichoepithelioma
- Syringoma
- Xanthoma

LABORATORY WORK-UP
- None

MANAGEMENT
- Comedo extraction
- Surgical excision
- Topical retinoids

SPECIFIC THERAPY
- Tretinoin 0.025% cream applied HS

CAVEATS AND PITFALLS
- Incomplete response to topical retinoids.

FIXED DRUG ERUPTION

ALTERNATE DISEASE NAME
- Fixed medication reaction
- Fixed eruption

HISTORY
- Onset 6–48 hours after dose of causative medication
- Common offenders include sulfonamides, nonsteroidal anti-inflammatory drugs, barbiturates, phenolphthalein & tetracycline
- Recurrence in the same site w/ re-administration of offending drug

PHYSICAL EXAMINATION
- Pruritus & burning, occasionally accompanied by fever at onset
- Begins as a few sharply demarcated, erythematous macules that rapidly become erythematous plaques, which heal w/ hyperpigmentation
- Occur most commonly on the lips in women & penis in men

DIFFERENTIAL DIAGNOSIS
- Contact dermatitis
- Herpes simplex virus infection
- Erythema multiforme
- Erythema migrans
- Chemical burn

- Bullous pemphigoid
- Lupus erythematosus
- Psoriasis
- Porphyria cutanea tarda
- Bullous disease of diabetes mellitus
- Postinflammatory hyperpigmentation
- Factitial disease

LABORATORY WORK-UP
- None

MANAGEMENT
- Discontinue use of offending medication

SPECIFIC THERAPY
- None

CAVEATS AND PITFALLS
- Postinflammatory hyperpigmentation may be permanent, even after stopping offending medication.

FOLLICULITIS

ALTERNATE DISEASE NAME
- None

HISTORY
- Gradually evolving red papules in hair-bearing areas
- May be asymptomatic or cause mild pain or pruritus
- Predisposing factors: staphylococcal nasal carriers, skin injuries, abrasions, surgical wounds, draining abscesses, skin occlusion for topical corticosteroid therapy, diabetes mellitus & immunosuppression

PHYSICAL EXAMINATION
- Primary lesion is a perifollicular papule or pustule, often appearing in grid-like pattern of multiple red papules and/or pustules on hair-bearing areas such as face, scalp, thighs, axilla & inguinal area
- Staphylococcal folliculitis
  - Follicular-based red papules & pustules
  - Caused by *Staphylococcus aureus*

- Hot tub folliculitis
  - Pruritic, edematous, erythematous papules or pustules in areas of skin occluded by a bathing suit
  - Caused by *Pseudomonas* organisms in tub or pool water
- *Pityrosporum* folliculitis
  - Pruritic acneform papules on upper back, chest, upper arms, neck, chin & sides of face
  - Caused by yeast forms of *Pityrosporum ovale*
- Fungal folliculitis
  - Affects the coarse hairs in the mustache & beard area in men
  - Caused by candidal species & dermatophytes

DIFFERENTIAL DIAGNOSIS
- Erythema toxicum
- Miliaria
- Insect bite reaction
- Pseudofolliculitis barbae
- Scabies
- Acne vulgaris
- Rosacea
- Perioral dermatitis
- Keratosis pilaris
- Acquired perforating disease
- Pemphigus foliaceus
- Darier disease
- Hailey-Hailey disease

LABORATORY WORK-UP
- Culture pustule contents for bacterial & fungal pathogens

MANAGEMENT
- Treatment of infection as per culture results
- Removal of inciting factors, such as tight-fitting clothing
- Systemic antibiotics as antiinflammatory or antibiotic agents

SPECIFIC THERAPY
- Tetracycline 500 mg PO BID indefinitely
- Doxycycline 50–100 mg PO BID indefinitely
- Minocycline 50–100 mg PO BID indefinitely

- Dapsone 25–100 mg PO QD indefinitely; use only after other agents have failed

CAVEATS AND PITFALLS
- Advise about possible gray discoloration of skin w/ prolonged minocycline use.
- Check CBC Q2–3 weeks for 10–12 weeks w/ dapsone to detect rare pancytopenia.

FOLLICULITIS DECALVANS

ALTERNATE DISEASE NAME
- None

HISTORY
- End result of various follicular inflammatory processes, including bacterial & inflammatory folliculitis
- Occurs in women after age 30 & in men from adolescence onward

PHYSICAL EXAMINATION
- Bogginess or induration of affected areas of the scalp or other hair-bearing sites
- Successive crops of pustules, often w/ subsequent scarring alopecia

DIFFERENTIAL DIAGNOSIS
- Dissecting folliculitis
- Lupus erythematosus
- Lichen planopilaris
- Kerion
- Pseudofolliculitis barbae
- Pseudopelade of Brocq
- Follicular degeneration syndrome
- Pemphigus vulgaris
- Pemphigus foliaceous
- Darier disease
- Hailey-Hailey disease

LABORATORY WORK-UP
- Bacterial culture of lesion contents

MANAGEMENT
- Treatment of infection only w/ positive cultures

SPECIFIC THERAPY
- None

CAVEATS AND PITFALLS
- None

FOX-FORDYCE DISEASE

ALTERNATE DISEASE NAME
- Fox-Fordyce syndrome
- Apocrine miliaria

HISTORY
- More common in women
- May first appear under conditions of heat, humidity & friction
- Significant pruritus, which may interfere w/ sleep

PHYSICAL EXAMINATION
- Pruritic, flesh-colored to reddish, smooth, dome-shaped, discrete, follicular or perifollicular papules
- Appears most commonly in axilla, but may affect periareolar, inframammary & pubic areas
- Anhidrosis in affected sites

DIFFERENTIAL DIAGNOSIS
- Folliculitis
- Hidradenitis suppurativa
- Pseudofolliculitis of axilla
- Miliaria
- Milia
- Follicular hamartomas

LABORATORY WORK-UP
- None

MANAGEMENT
- Topical retinoids
- Surgical excision of axilla
- Liposuction-assisted curettage

SPECIFIC THERAPY
- Tretinoin 0.025% cream applied HS

CAVEATS AND PITFALLS
- Incomplete response to topical retinoids.

FURUNCLE

ALTERNATE DISEASE NAME
- Boil
- Abscess
- Carbuncle (aggregation of several furuncles)

HISTORY
- Hard red papule that softens & becomes more painful over several days

PHYSICAL EXAMINATION
- Occurs only in hair-bearing areas, most commonly on neck, face, axillae, buttocks & thighs
- Begins as red, painful papule or nodule, which enlarges over a few days
- Spontaneous rupture yields pus & necrotic debris.
- Resolution w/ post-inflammatory hyperpigmentation

DIFFERENTIAL DIAGNOSIS
- Inflamed epidermoid cyst
- Hidradenitis suppurativa
- Folliculitis
- Acne vulgaris
- Foreign body reaction
- Myiasis
- Factitial disease

LABORATORY WORK-UP
- Culture of abscess contents for bacterial pathogens

MANAGEMENT
- Incision & drainage if there is fluctuant material
- Warm compresses applied for 30 minutes QID
- Systemic antibiotics

SPECIFIC THERAPY
- Dicloxacillin 250–500 mg PO QID for 7–10 days
- Cephalexin 250–500 mg PO QID for 7 days
- Azithromycin 500 mg PO QD for 3 days

CAVEATS AND PITFALLS
- Consider hidradenitis suppurativa if lesions are in axilla or groin area.

GIANOTTI-CROSTI SYNDROME

ALTERNATE DISEASE NAME
- Papular acrodermatitis of childhood
- Papular infantile acrodermatitis
- Infantile papular acrodermatitis
- Infantile lichenoid acrodermatitis
- Acrodermatitis papulosa eruptiva infantilis
- Acrodermatitis papulosa infantum

HISTORY
- Most common in children
- Prodrome of mild constitutional symptoms
- Respiratory infection may precede skin disease

PHYSICAL EXAMINATION
- Pale, pink to flesh-colored papules localized symmetrically over extremities, buttocks & face
- Papules may be smooth-topped, polished, w/ mild pruritus
- Complete resolution in several months

DIFFERENTIAL DIAGNOSIS
- Pityriasis rosea
- Pityriasis lichenoides
- Atopic dermatitis
- Lichen planus
- Drug eruption
- Langerhans cell histiocytosis
- Polymorphous light eruption
- Sarcoidosis
- Granuloma annulare
- Scabies

- Flat warts
- Lichen nitidus

LABORATORY WORK-UP
- None

MANAGEMENT
- None

SPECIFIC THERAPY
- None

CAVEATS AND PITFALLS
- None

GLOMUS TUMOR

ALTERNATE DISEASE NAME
- Glomangioma

HISTORY
- Multiple tumors occur on familial basis
- Paroxysmal pain, exacerbated by pressure or temperature changes, especially cold temperatures

PHYSICAL EXAMINATION
- Solitary glomus tumor
  - Blanchable blue or purple papule, usually located in acral areas, especially subungual areas of fingers & toes
- Multiple glomus tumors
  - Pain is usually minimal
  - Regional variant: blue to purple, compressible papules or nodules that are grouped & limited to a specific area, most commonly over an extremity
  - Disseminated form: multiple lesions distributed over the body w/ no specific grouping
- Congenital plaque-like form: grouped papules coalescing into indurated plaques or clusters of discrete nodules

DIFFERENTIAL DIAGNOSIS
- Angioleiomyoma
- Angiolipoma

- Arteriovenous malformation
- Blue nevus
- Hemangioma, including tufted angioma
- Melanoma
- Spiradenoma
- Kaposi's sarcoma
- Blue rubber bleb nevus
- Neurilemmoma

LABORATORY WORK-UP
- Lesional biopsy

MANAGEMENT
- Solitary glomus tumor: surgical excision
- Multiple glomus tumors: surgical removal for cosmetic reasons only

SPECIFIC THERAPY
- See "Management"

CAVEATS AND PITFALLS
- None

GLUCAGONOMA SYNDROME

ALTERNATE DISEASE NAME
- Necrolytic migratory erythema

HISTORY
- Nonspecific complaints such as weight loss, diarrhea & stomatitis
- New-onset diabetes mellitus

PHYSICAL EXAMINATION
- Necrolytic migratory erythema
  - Found anywhere on the body, but most common in perineum, buttocks, groin, lower abdomen & lower extremities
  - Eruption begins as a pruritic or painful, erythematous patch that blisters centrally, erodes, crusts over & heals w/ hyperpigmentation.
  - Annular papules w/ confluence into plaques in severely affected areas

- Mucocutaneous findings include atrophic glossitis, cheilosis, dystrophic nails & buccal mucosal inflammation

DIFFERENTIAL DIAGNOSIS
- Acrodermatitis enteropathica
- Hailey-Hailey disease
- Darier disease
- Candidiasis
- Paraneoplastic pemphigus
- Pellagra
- Kwashiorkor

LABORATORY WORK-UP
- Serum glucagon, serum insulin, gastrin & vasoactive intestinal peptide levels
- Glucose tolerance test
- Nutritional profile consisting of amino acid, zinc & essential fatty acid levels
- CT of abdomen
- Celiac axis angiography

MANAGEMENT
- Surgical resection of tumor, if localized
- In the absence of tumor, treat underlying cause

SPECIFIC THERAPY
- See "Management"

CAVEATS AND PITFALLS
- None

GONOCOCCEMIA

ALTERNATE DISEASE NAME
- Gonococcal dermatitis-arthritis syndrome
- Disseminated gonococcal infection

HISTORY
- More common in women, often w/ asymptomatic infection

- Risk factors: high sexual activity, lower socioeconomic status, ethnic minority, male homosexual, drug use, lower educational level, past history of other sexually transmitted diseases

PHYSICAL EXAMINATION
- Disseminated disease generally follows primary genital infection by several days to 2 weeks
- Fever; myalgias; tenosynovitis; monoarticular septic arthritis, affecting large, weight-bearing joints
- Acral palpable purpuric papules & pustules, usually relatively few in number

DIFFERENTIAL DIAGNOSIS
- Meningococcemia or other infectious causes of septic vasculitis
- Lupus erythematosus
- Reiter syndrome
- Infective endocarditis
- Cryoglobulinemia

LABORATORY WORK-UP
- Culture for *N. gonorrhoeae* from mucosal sites, including pharynx, urethra, cervix or rectum

MANAGEMENT
- Systemic antibiotics
- Treat for presumed chlamydial infection also

SPECIFIC THERAPY
- Ceftriaxone 1 g IM or IV q24h for 3 days or until 24 hours after symptomatic improvement
- Complete 7-day course w/ ciprofloxacin 500 mg PO twice daily or cefixime 400 mg PO twice daily or azithromycin 500 mg PO per day
- Concurrent therapy for presumed chlamydia w/ doxycycline 100 mg PO BID for 7 days

CAVEATS AND PITFALLS
- Evaluate for other sexually transmitted diseases.

GRAFT-VERSUS-HOST DISEASE

ALTERNATE DISEASE NAME
- None

HISTORY
- Incidence higher in recipients of allogeneic hematopoietic cells than in pts receiving syngeneic or autologous hematopoietic cells
- Onset of acute GVHD 10–30 days after transplantation
- Onset of chronic GVHD after day 100 post-transplantation
- Chronic GVHD usually evolves from acute GVHD but may occur de novo

PHYSICAL EXAMINATION
- Acute GVHD
  - Eruption begins as faint, tender, erythematous macules, often centered around hair follicles
  - As disease progresses, more erythematous macules appear & coalesce to form confluent plaques or papules
  - Subepidermal bullae occasionally occur
- Chronic GVHD
  - Violaceous lichenified papules, often on ventral skin surfaces, very similar to those of lichen planus
  - Lacy white plaques on buccal mucosa
  - Sclerodermatous changes, including scattered sclerotic plaques & widespread disease resulting in ulcerations, joint contractures & esophageal dysmotility

DIFFERENTIAL DIAGNOSIS
- Acute GVHD
  - Erythema multiforme
  - Drug eruption
  - Stevens-Johnson syndrome/toxic epidermal necrolysis
  - Eruption of lymphocyte recovery
- Chronic GVHD
  - Scleroderma
  - Lichen planus
  - Lichenoid drug eruption
  - Lupus erythematosus

LABORATORY WORK-UP
- Lesional biopsy
- Liver function studies
- Stool & blood cultures if there is diarrhea

MANAGEMENT
- Acute GVHD
  - Systemic corticosteroids for symptomatic disease
  - Extracorporeal photochemotherapy
- Chronic GVHD
  - Photochemotherapy or extracorporeal photochemotherapy Narrowband UVB phototherapy
  - Methotrexate
  - Hydroxychloroquine
  - Systemic retinoids

SPECIFIC THERAPY
- Acute form
  - Prednisone 1 mg/kg PO QAM
- Chronic form
  - Methotrexate 7.5–25 mg PO Q 7 days
  - Hydroxychloroquine 200 mg PO BID
  - Acitretin 25–75 mg PO QD

CAVEATS AND PITFALLS
- Presence of chronic GVHD is poor prognostic sign.

GRANULAR CELL TUMOR

ALTERNATE DISEASE NAME
- Granular cell myoblastoma
- Granular cell schwannoma
- Granular cell neuroma
- Granular cell neurofibroma

HISTORY
- Insidious onset & slow growth of asymptomatic papule or nodule

PHYSICAL EXAMINATION
- Discrete, asymptomatic, firm, flesh-colored papule or nodule, occurring on tongue, head & neck region or dorsal aspect of forearms

DIFFERENTIAL DIAGNOSIS
- Neurofibroma
- Fibroma
- Squamous cell carcinoma
- Wart
- Dermatofibroma
- Epidermoid cyst

LABORATORY WORK-UP
- Lesional biopsy

MANAGEMENT
- Surgical excision

SPECIFIC THERAPY
- Elliptical excision

CAVEATS AND PITFALLS
- None

GRANULOMA FACIALE

ALTERNATE DISEASE NAME
- Facial granuloma
- Granuloma faciale eosinophilicum
- Granuloma faciale w/ eosinophilia

HISTORY
- Insidious onset of asymptomatic skin lesion

PHYSICAL EXAMINATION
- Solitary or multiple, sharply marginated, red or violaceous papules or nodules, usually on face but occasionally on trunk or upper extremities
- Surface may have telangiectasias and/or enlarged follicular orifices

DIFFERENTIAL DIAGNOSIS
- Benign lymphocytic infiltrate (Jessner)
- Lupus erythematosus
- Lymphoma

- Sarcoidosis
- Granuloma annulare
- Mycosis fungoides
- Fixed drug eruption
- Leprosy
- Lupus vulgaris
- Foreign body granuloma

LABORATORY WORK-UP
- Lesional biopsy

MANAGEMENT
- Intralesional corticosteroids
- Sulfones

SPECIFIC THERAPY
- Triamcinolone 3–4 mg/mL intralesional
- Dapsone 25–100 mg PO QD

CAVEATS AND PITFALLS
- Check CBC Q2–3 weeks for 10–12 weeks w/ dapsone to detect rare pancytopenia.
  - Obtain baseline G6PD level before starting dapsone.

GRANULOMA INGUINALE

ALTERNATE DISEASE NAME
- Donovanosis

HISTORY
- Sexually transmitted disease w/ incubation period 1 week to 3 months

PHYSICAL EXAMINATION
- Occurs on glans penis & scrotum in men, labia minora, mons veneris & fourchette in women, w/ rare cervical involvement
- Soft, red papules or nodules arising at site of inoculation
- Lesions ulcerate & develop red, granulating, friable, spreading plaques & nodules
- Ulcers w/ clean, friable bases & distinct, raised, rolled margins
- Autoinoculation causes lesions on adjacent skin

- Occasional hypertrophic or verrucous plaques, w/ formation of large, vegetating masses resembling genital warts
- Swelling of external genitalia occurs in later-stage lesions

DIFFERENTIAL DIAGNOSIS
- Syphilis
- Lymphogranuloma venereum
- Herpes simplex virus infection
- Squamous cell carcinoma
- Lichen sclerosus

LABORATORY WORK-UP
- Crush preparation of lesional tissue examined w/ Wright-Giemsa or Warthin-Starry stain, looking for Donovan bodies

MANAGEMENT
- Systemic antibiotics

SPECIFIC THERAPY
- Trimethoprim/sulfamethoxazole DS capsule BID for at least 3 weeks
- Doxycycline 100 mg PO BID for at least 3 weeks

CAVEATS AND PITFALLS
- Check for other sexually transmitted diseases.

HAIRY TONGUE

ALTERNATE DISEASE NAME
- Black hairy tongue
- Lingua nigra
- Lingua villosa
- Lingua villosa nigra

HISTORY
- Gradual onset of asymptomatic tongue lesion
- Associated w/ smoking, poor oral hygiene

PHYSICAL EXAMINATION
- Elongation of filiform papillae on dorsal surface of tongue
- Brown, black or reddish discoloration of tongue plaque

DIFFERENTIAL DIAGNOSIS
- Candidiasis
- Lichen planus
- Oral hairy leukoplakia

LABORATORY WORK-UP
- None

MANAGEMENT
- Physical tongue debridement by mechanical removal of elongated papillae by brushing tongue w/ a toothbrush or using a tongue blade
- Improve oral hygiene, including discontinuing smoking

SPECIFIC THERAPY
- Destruction by electrodesiccation & curettage

CAVEATS AND PITFALLS
- None

HERPES GESTATIONIS

ALTERNATE DISEASE NAME
- Pemphigoid gestationis
- Autoimmune dermatosis of pregnancy
- Pregnancy-associated autoimmune disease

HISTORY
- Eruption occurs during 2d & 3d trimesters of pregnancy or immediately after delivery
- Disease activity often remits within days after parturition, but some pts experience persistent disease activity that lasts months or years
- May recur with resumption of menses, use of oral contraception & subsequent pregnancies

PHYSICAL EXAMINATION
- Presents as intensely pruritic erythematous urticarial patches & plaques, often periumbilical
- Lesions evolve into tense vesicles & bullae, spreading peripherally, often sparing face, palms, soles & mucous membranes

DIFFERENTIAL DIAGNOSIS
- Bullous pemphigoid
- Linear IgA bullous dermatosis
- Dermatitis herpetiformis
- Pruritic urticarial papules & plaques of pregnancy (PUPPP)
- Herpes simplex virus infection
- Prurigo gestationis of Besnier
- Pruritic folliculitis of pregnancy

LABORATORY WORK-UP
- Skin biopsy for routine light microscopy
- Skin biopsy of noninvolved perilesional skin for direct immuno-fluorescence

MANAGEMENT
- Mild disease: topical corticosteroids
- Severe disease: systemic corticosteroids

SPECIFIC THERAPY
- Mild disease: fluocinonide 0.05% cream applied BID
- Severe disease: prednisone 1 mg/kg PO QAM until no further vesiculation; then slow taper over several weeks

CAVEATS AND PITFALLS
- If prednisone is to be used for >21 days per course of therapy, obtain baseline chest radiograph, TB skin test & bone mineral density determination.

HERPES SIMPLEX VIRUS INFECTION

ALTERNATE DISEASE NAME
- None

HISTORY
- Neonatal infection begins within 24 hours of birth w/ signs of serious systemic illness
- Primary infection has prodrome of constitutional signs & symptoms
- Most clinical skin infections represent re-infection (secondary infection)

PHYSICAL EXAMINATION
- Neonatal infection
  - Grouped vesicles on erythematous base in only 20% of children w/ disseminated disease
  - New lesions form adjacent to old vesicles, coalescing into larger, irregular vesicles or bullae
  - Manifestations of illness represent the organ systems involved (ie, CNS, lungs, GI tract, heart, kidneys); skin vesicles develop from an erythematous base
- Acute gingivostomatitis
  - Most frequent clinical presentation of first-episode, primary HSV infection
  - Gingivitis w/ markedly swollen, erythematous, bleeding gums; occasional increased drooling noted in infants
  - Vesicular lesions occur on tongue, buccal mucosa & palate, w/ extension to lips & face
  - Tender submandibular or cervical adenopathy
  - Disease course from 3–7 days
- Recurrent orolabial herpetic infection (herpes labialis)
  - Prodrome of pain, tingling, burning or itching, usually lasting up to 6 hours
  - Vesicular rash in crops of 3–5 vesicles, frequently arising near vermillion border
  - Recurrences often associated w/ febrile illnesses, local trauma, sun exposure or menstruation
- Primary genital infections
  - May have severe constitutional symptoms: fever, malaise, myalgias & occasional headache
  - Vesicular rash w/ lesions progressing to pustules or painful ulcerative papules
  - Process may last up to 3 weeks
  - Painful inguinal lymphadenopathy
  - Dysuria & vaginal discharge
- Recurrent genital infections
  - Vulvar irritation and/or ulcerating or vesicular lesions
  - Symptoms more severe in females than in males
  - Recurrent infections in males sometimes present w/ vesicular lesions on shaft of penis
  - Local symptoms of recurrence include pain, itching & dysuria

- Localized eye infection
  - Presents w/ conjunctival injection & a watery discharge
  - Characteristic dendritic lesions on fluorescein staining of cornea
- CNS infection
  - Encephalitis possible manifestation of primary or recurrent infection
  - Other sequelae include aseptic meningitis, transverse myelitis
- Herpetic whitlow (infection of a digit)
  - Presents w/ acute onset of edema, erythema & localized pain & tenderness in the finger
  - Associated fever & regional adenopathy

LABORATORY WORK-UP
- Use only if diagnosis is not established clinically
  - Tzanck preparation, looking for multinucleated giant cells
  - Viral culture
  - Direct fluorescence antibody (DFA) testing

MANAGEMENT
- Systemic antiviral agents for immunocompromised individuals
- Systemic antiviral agents for prophylaxis w/ frequent recurrences

SPECIFIC THERAPY
- Acute infection
  - Famciclovir 500 mg PO BID for 7 days
  - Valacyclovir 100 mg PO BID for 7 days
- Viral prophylaxis
  - Famciclovir 250 mg PO BID
  - Valacyclovir 500 mg PO QD

CAVEATS AND PITFALLS
- Recurrent erythema multiforme may occur w/ each episode in some pts.

HERPES ZOSTER

ALTERNATE DISEASE NAME
- Shingles
- Zoster

HISTORY
- Mild constitutional symptoms as baseline
- Prodromal pain and/or dysesthesia for 1–5 days before onset of eruption

PHYSICAL EXAMINATION
- Early patchy erythema in dermatomal area of involvement, w/ regional lymphadenopathy
- Unilateral, grouped vesicles on erythematous base, w/ severe local pain
- Vesicles initially clear, but eventually become pustular, rupture & form crusts
- Scarring occurs if deeper skin layers are traumatized by scratching, secondary infection or other complications
- Zoster oticus (geniculate zoster, zoster auris, Ramsay-Hunt syndrome, Hunt syndrome)
  - Starts w/ otalgia & herpetiform vesicles on external ear canal, w/ or w/out features of facial paralysis
  - Auditory symptoms (eg, deafness) & vestibular symptoms may be present
- Disseminated zoster
  - Generalized eruption of >15–25 extra-dermatomal vesicles, occurring 5–14 days after onset of dermatomal disease
  - More common in elderly, hospitalized or immunocompromised pts
  - Often an indication of depressed cell-mediated immunity caused by various underlying clinical situations, including malignancies, radiation therapy, cancer chemotherapy, organ transplants & chronic use of systemic corticosteroids
  - May have involvement of lungs & CNS

DIFFERENTIAL DIAGNOSIS
- Varicella
- Herpes simplex virus infection
- Impetigo
- Candidiasis
- Erysipelas
- Cellulitis
- Bullous pemphigoid
- Pemphigus vulgaris
- Contact dermatitis

- Urticaria
- Photoallergic reaction
- Folliculitis
- Insect bite reaction
- Brachioradial pruritus

LABORATORY WORK-UP
- Use only if diagnosis is not established clinically
- Tzanck preparation, looking for multinucleated giant cells
- Viral culture
- Direct fluorescence antibody (DFA) testing

MANAGEMENT
- Systemic antiviral agents for pts over age 50 or immunocompromised individuals
- Aggressive pain mgt, including narcotic analgesics

SPECIFIC THERAPY
- Acute infection
  - Famciclovir 500 mg PO TID for 7 days
  - Valacyclovir 100 mg PO TID for 7 days
- Postherpetic neuralgia
  - Capsaicin 0.75% cream applied 4 or 5 times per day; advise about burning sensation w/ each application
  - Tricyclic antidepressants, such as amitriptyline, 25–100 mg PO daily
  - Gabapentin: 300–2,400 mg PO daily

CAVEATS AND PITFALLS
- Zoster oticus may be mistaken for eczema, Ménière disease, Bell palsy, cerebrovascular accident or abscess of ear.
- Little or no benefit of antiviral therapy in pts under age 50 years.

HIDRADENITIS SUPPURATIVA

ALTERNATE DISEASE NAME
- Suppurative hidradenitis
- Apocrine acne
- Apocrinitis

HISTORY

- Hirsutism & obesity common findings among affected women
- Insidious onset w/ early symptoms & signs of pruritus, erythema & local hyperhidrosis

PHYSICAL EXAMINATION

- Painful, tender, red papules & nodules in axillae, groin area, nipples & buttocks, which heal w/ fibrosis & eventual recurrence in adjacent area
- May evolve into fluctuant abscesses, which may become infected
- Dermal contractures & rope-like scars
- Multiple abscesses & sinus tracts form a subcutaneous honeycomb
- Double-headed comedos in area of nodules & papules
- Associated arthropathy w/ variable clinical features ranging from asymmetric pauciarticular arthritis to a symmetric polyarthritis or polyarthralgia syndrome

DIFFERENTIAL DIAGNOSIS

- Staphylococcal abscess
- Infected or inflamed epidermoid cyst
- Furuncle or carbuncle
- Granuloma inguinale
- Lymphogranuloma venereum
- Actinomycosis
- Bartholin cyst
- Crohn disease
- Tuberculosis
- Tularemia
- Ulcerative colitis

LABORATORY WORK-UP

- Bacterial culture of fluctuant nodule

MANAGEMENT

- Wide surgical excision, preferably taking as much apocrine gland-bearing skin as possible
- Early disease
- Surgical techniques include incision & drainage; exteriorization, curettage; electrocoagulation of sinus tracts & simple excision

- Intralesional corticosteroids to inflamed nodules
- Systemic antibiotics as anti-inflammatory agents
- Sulfones
- Systemic retinoids

SPECIFIC THERAPY
- Triamcinolone 3–5 mg/kg intralesionally to inflamed nodules
- Tetracycline 500 mg PO BID
- Doxycycline 100 mg PO BID
- Minocycline 100 mg PO BID
- Isotretinoin 1 mg/kg PO QD for 5–6 months
- Dapsone 25–100 mg PO QD

CAVEATS AND PITFALLS
- Surgery most effective if performed early in course of disease.
- Minor benefit of antibiotics used as antiinflammatory agents.
- Check CBC Q2–3 weeks for 10–12 weeks w/ dapsone to detect rare pancytopenia.
- Absolute contraindication of isotretinoin in pregnant women.

HIDROCYSTOMA

ALTERNATE DISEASE NAME
- Cystadenoma
- Sudoriferous cyst

HISTORY
- Slowly enlarging, asymptomatic lesion(s) on face

PHYSICAL EXAMINATION
- Translucent papule or nodule
- Predilection for eyelid, particularly inner canthus
- Contains thin, clear or brownish fluid

DIFFERENTIAL DIAGNOSIS
- Basal cell carcinoma
- Epidermoid cyst
- Syringoma
- Milium

LABORATORY WORK-UP
- Biopsy to confirm diagnosis

MANAGEMENT
- Destructive treatment modalities
- Punch, shave or elliptical excision

SPECIFIC THERAPY
- Incision & drainage, followed by surgical destruction of the wall by light electrodesiccation & curettage

CAVEATS AND PITFALLS
- None

HIDROTIC ECTODERMAL DYSPLASIA

ALTERNATE DISEASE NAME
- Hereditary hidrotic ectodermal dysplasia
- Clouston's disease

HISTORY
- Familial clustering
- Present at birth

PHYSICAL EXAMINATION
- Dystrophic nails
- Sparse, thin, fragile hair
- Hyperkeratosis of palms & soles
- Normal sweat function; skin dryness

DIFFERENTIAL DIAGNOSIS
- Anhidrotic ectodermal dysplasia
- Dyskeratosis congenita
- Pachonychia congenita
- Basan syndrome
- Chondroectodermal dysplasia

LABORATORY WORK-UP
- None

MANAGEMENT
- Dental prophylaxis
- Ocular lubrication

SPECIFIC THERAPY
- None

CAVEATS AND PITFALLS
- None

HISTOPLASMOSIS

ALTERNATE DISEASE NAME
- Darling's disease

HISTORY
- Travel or residence in an endemic area or activities involving bats or birds; endemic areas include central river valleys in the midwestern & south-central USA

PHYSICAL EXAMINATION
- Acute pulmonary infection
  - Usually asymptomatic
  - With symptomatic disease, fever, headache, malaise, myalgia, abdominal pain & chills
  - Severe dyspnea may occur w/ exposure to large inoculum
  - Nonspecific signs of infection include erythema nodosum & erythema multiforme
- Chronic pulmonary disease
  - Appears mostly in pts w/ underlying pulmonary disease
  - Cough, weight loss, fevers & malaise
  - If cavitations are present, hemoptysis, sputum production & increasing dyspnea
- Progressive disseminated disease
  - Occurs mostly in immunocompromised pts
  - Skin lesions start as small papules that ulcerate
  - Oropharyngeal ulcers involve buccal mucosa, tongue, gingiva & larynx

DIFFERENTIAL DIAGNOSIS
- Bacterial or mycoplasma pneumonia
- North American blastomycosis
- Coccidioidomycosis
- Tuberculosis

- Sarcoidosis
- Aspergillosis
- Lymphoma
- Lung cancer

LABORATORY WORK-UP
- Sputum & blood cultures
- Serologies for *H. capsulatum* (IgG & IgM antibodies)
- Chest radiograph
- Lesional skin biopsy

MANAGEMENT
- Mildly symptomatic or prolonged acute pulmonary histoplasmosis: oral antifungal therapy
- Progressive disease, particularly w/ meningitis: amphotericin B

SPECIFIC THERAPY
- Ketoconazole 200–400 mg PO QD for 6–12 months
- Itraconazole 200–400 mg PO QD for 6–12 months
- Amphotericin B 0.7–1 mg/kg per day IV to a total dose of 35 mg/kg

CAVEATS AND PITFALLS
- No therapy indicated for asymptomatic disease or for cutaneous disease as sole sign of dissemination.

HOT TUB FOLLICULITIS

ALTERNATE DISEASE NAME
- *Pseudomonas* folliculitis
- Hot tub dermatitis
- Whirlpool folliculitis
- Splash rash

HISTORY
- Minor trauma from vigorous rubbing w/ sponges, etc may facilitate entry of organisms into skin
- Hot water, high pH (>7.8) & low chlorine level are predisposing factors
- Onset usually about 48 hours after exposure to contaminated water

PHYSICAL EXAMINATION
- Follicular papules, vesicles & pustules, which may be crusted, on exposed skin, but usually sparing face, neck, palms & soles
- Lesions evolve to erythematous papules & pustules & clear spontaneously w/out scarring in 2–10 days
- May have postinflammatory hyperpigmented macules
- Occasional mild accompanying constitutional symptoms & signs

DIFFERENTIAL DIAGNOSIS
- Inflammatory folliculitis
- Insect bite reaction
- Staphylococcal folliculitis
- Grover's disease
- Pityriasis lichenoides et varioliformis acuta
- Scabies

LABORATORY WORK-UP
- Culture follicular pustule if there is doubt about diagnosis

MANAGEMENT
- No effective therapy for this self-limited condition

SPECIFIC THERAPY
- None

CAVEATS AND PITFALLS
- May have postinflammatory hyperpigmentation

HYPEREOSINOPHILIC SYNDROME

ALTERNATE DISEASE NAME
- Idiopathic hypereosinophilic syndrome

HISTORY
- Early symptoms include fatigue, cough, dyspnea, myalgia, angioedema fever, sweating & pruritus
- Presenting complaint can vary depending on organ involved

PHYSICAL EXAMINATION
- Cutaneous findings

- ➤ Pruritus; angioedema, urticaria, often w/ dermatographism
- ➤ Erythematous, pruritic papules, plaques & nodules, w/ or w/out ulceration
- Cardiac findings include chest pain, dyspnea & orthopnea
- Hematologic changes include splenomegaly & thromboses
- Neurologic findings include encephalopathy; cerebrovascular accidents & transient ischemic episodes
- Pulmonary findings include chronic, persistent cough, dyspnea from congestive heart failure or pleural effusion & pulmonary fibrosis
- Rheumatologic findings include arthralgias & myalgias & Raynaud phenomenon
- GI findings include abdominal pain, nausea & diarrhea & hepatomegaly

DIFFERENTIAL DIAGNOSIS
- Angiolymphoid hyperplasia w/ eosinophilia
- Atopic dermatitis
- Drug reaction
- Lupus erythematosus
- Parasitic infection
- Malignancy w/ secondary eosinophilia
- Churg-Strauss syndrome
- Eosinophilic fasciitis
- Eosinophilia-myalgia syndrome

LABORATORY WORK-UP
- CBC, looking for peripheral eosinophilia & possible anemia
- Serum immunoglobulin levels, looking for elevated IgE levels
- Urinalysis, looking for proteinuria, hematuria, albuminuria, and/or hyaline casts

MANAGEMENT
- Systemic corticosteroids
- Cytotoxic drugs or antimetabolites in pts who fail corticosteroids
- Photochemotherapy for symptomatic control of extensive skin eruption & pruritus

SPECIFIC THERAPY
- Prednisone 1 mg/kg PO QAM indefinitely

- Aggressive disease unresponsive to corticosteroids
  - Hydroxyurea 20–30 mg/kg PO per day
  - Vincristine 1–2 mg IV every 2 weeks
  - Chlorambucil pulse of 4–10 mg/m^2 per day PO for 4 days every other month
  - Bone marrow transplantation for life-threatening disease

CAVEATS AND PITFALLS
- If prednisone is to be used for >21 days per course of therapy, obtain baseline chest radiograph, TB skin test & bone mineral density determination.
  - May be associated w/ myeloproliferative disorders

HYPERIMMUNOGLOBULIN E SYNDROME

ALTERNATE DISEASE NAME
- Hyper IgE syndrome
- Job syndrome
- Job's syndrome

HISTORY
- Moderate to severe, pruritic, eczematous skin eruptions in early life
- Multiple infections from infancy

PHYSICAL EXAMINATION
- Coarse facies
- Early nonspecific papular or pustular eruption, favoring scalp, proximal flexures & buttocks
- Eczematous eruption
- Recurrent staphylococcal abscesses, w/out pain, heat, or redness
- Other infections, including cellulitis, recurrent bronchitis, chronic mucocutaneous candidiasis & onychomycosis
- Skeletal abnormalities, including frequent painless bone fractures, scoliosis & hyperextensible joints

DIFFERENTIAL DIAGNOSIS
- Atopic dermatitis
- Chronic mucocutaneous candidiasis

- Recurrent folliculitis
- Staphylococcal carriage state w/ recurrent skin infections
- Wiskott-Aldrich syndrome
- DiGeorge syndrome
- Chronic granulomatous disease
- Common variable immunodeficiency
- X-linked hypogammaglobulinemia
- Leukocyte adhesion deficiency

LABORATORY WORK-UP
- CBC, looking for peripheral eosinophilia
- Serum immunoglobulin levels, looking for elevated IgE levels
- Pulmonary imaging (chest radiograph, CT)

MANAGEMENT
- Antibiotics for bacterial infections
- Prophylaxis w/ antiseptic scrubs, ascorbic acid & cimetidine

SPECIFIC THERAPY
- Active bacterial infection
  - Adults: nafcillin 500–2,000 mg IV q6h for 1–5 days, depending on therapeutic response; then dicloxacillin 500 mg PO 4 times daily for 10–21 days, depending on therapeutic response
  - Children: nafcillin 100–200 mg/kg IV per day in 4 divided doses for 1–5 days, depending on therapeutic response; then dicloxacillin 250 mg PO QID for 10–21 days, depending on therapeutic response
- Incision & drainage of fluctuant abscesses
- Active candidiasis
  - Fluconazole 150 mg PO QD for 1–3 weeks
  - Cyclosporine 3–5 mg/kg PO QD
- Prophylaxis
  - Cimetidine 20–40 mg/kg PO 3 or 4 times per day
  - Ascorbic acid 500 mg PO per day
  - Antibacterial soaps used 1 or 2 times per day

CAVEATS AND PITFALLS
- None

HYPOMELANOSIS OF ITO

ALTERNATE DISEASE NAME
- Incontinentia pigmenti achromians

HISTORY
- Present at birth
- Congenital abnormalities, mental retardation & seizures may be associated

PHYSICAL EXAMINATION
- Asymmetric, hypopigmented or white macules coalescing to form reticulated patches along lines of Blaschko
- Patches & macules may cover >2 dermatomes & on both sides of body

DIFFERENTIAL DIAGNOSIS
- Incontinentia pigmenti
- Nevoid hypermelanosis
- Nevus depigmentosus
- Congenital nevocellular nevus
- Postinflammatory hyperpigmentation

LABORATORY WORK-UP
- None

MANAGEMENT
- Evaluate for neurologic dysfunction if there are localizing signs & symptoms

SPECIFIC THERAPY
- None

CAVEATS AND PITFALLS
- No work-up required if there are no localizing signs of neurologic disease.

ICHTHYOSIS VULGARIS

ALTERNATE DISEASE NAME
- Common ichthyosis
- Autosomal dominant ichthyosis

- Hereditary ichthyosis vulgaris
- Fish skin ichthyosis
- Ichthyosis simplex
- Xeroderma
- Pityriasis vulgaris

HISTORY
- Familial involvement
- Disease worsens w/ age
- Improvement in summer or in warm climate

PHYSICAL EXAMINATION
- Symmetrical, variable scaling
- Small, fine, irregular & polygonal scales, often curling at edges to give skin a rough feel
- Most scaling occurs on extensor surfaces of extremities, w/ sharp demarcation between normal flexural folds & surrounding affected areas
- Lower extremities generally more affected than upper extremities; on trunk, scaling often more pronounced on back than abdomen
- Palmoplantar thickening & hyperlinearity
- Sparing of flexural folds & face

DIFFERENTIAL DIAGNOSIS
- X-linked ichthyosis
- Xerosis
- Acquired ichthyosis
- Atopic dermatitis
- Lamellar ichthyosis
- Sarcoidosis
- Dermatophytosis

LABORATORY WORK-UP
- None

MANAGEMENT
- Keratolytic agents
- Emollients

SPECIFIC THERAPY
- Keratolytics such as salicylic acid, glycolic acid or urea applied BID

CAVEATS AND PITFALLS
- Emollients mask the scale but do not remove it.

ID REACTION

ALTERNATE DISEASE NAME
- Autoeczematization
- Autosensitization

HISTORY
- Preceded by exacerbation of preexisting dermatitis
- Underlying conditions include dermatophyte infection, mycobacterial infection, viral or bacterial infection, contact dermatitis, stasis dermatitis or other eczematous processes

PHYSICAL EXAMINATION
- Acute onset of an extremely pruritic, symmetrical, erythematous, papular or papulovesicular eruption
- Vesicles may be present on hands or feet
- Eruption occurs at sites distant from primary dermatosis

DIFFERENTIAL DIAGNOSIS
- Atopic dermatitis
- Stasis dermatitis
- Seborrheic dermatitis
- Contact dermatitis
- Dyshidrotic eczema
- Dermatophytosis
- Scabies
- Gianotti-Crosti syndrome
- Pityriasis lichenoides et varioliformis acuta
- Drug eruption
- Folliculitis

LABORATORY WORK-UP
- None

MANAGEMENT
- Systemic corticosteroids
- Topical corticosteroids

SPECIFIC THERAPY
- Prednisone 1 mg/kg PO QAM for 7–14 days
- Triamcinolone 0.1% cream applied BID

CAVEATS AND PITFALLS
- Prednisone should be used for a maximum of 21 days per course.
- Clearing the primary dermatosis will clear the id reaction.

INCONTINENTIA PIGMENTI

ALTERNATE DISEASE NAME
- Bloch-Sulzberger syndrome
- Bloch-Siemens syndrome

HISTORY
- Present at birth, although not always w/ stage 1 findings

PHYSICAL EXAMINATION
- Cutaneous changes
    - Stage 1: linear, red papules & vesicles grouped on an erythematous base, mainly on extremities
    - Stage 2: linear, verrucous plaques on an erythematous base
    - Stage 3: streaks & whorls of brown or slate-gray pigmentation along lines of Blaschko, particularly on trunk
    - Stage 4: hypopigmented, atrophic, reticulated patches, mostly on lower extremities; lusterless, thin hair; nail dystrophy, ranging from mild pitting or ridging of the nail plate to severely thickened abnormally ridged nails; dental abnormalities
- Ocular findings include retinal detachment; proliferative retinopathy, fibrovascular retrolental membrane, cataracts & atrophy of the ciliary body
- Neurologic findings include seizures, developmental delay, mental retardation, ataxia, spasticity; microcephaly, cerebral atrophy, hypoplasia of the corpus callosum & periventricular cerebral edema

DIFFERENTIAL DIAGNOSIS
- Stage 1
  - Erythema toxicum
  - Bullous impetigo
  - Herpes simplex virus infection
  - Varicella
  - Epidermolysis bullosa
  - Bullous mastocytosis
  - Epidermolytic hyperkeratosis
- Stage 2
  - Linear epidermal nevus
  - Lichen striatus
  - X-linked dominant chondrodysplasia punctata
- Stage 3
  - Linear & whorled nevoid hypermelanosis
  - Dermatopathia pigmentosa reticularis
  - Naegeli-Franceschetti-Jadassohn syndrome
- Stage 4
  - Hypomelanosis of Ito
  - Focal dermal hypoplasia syndrome

LABORATORY WORK-UP
- Head MRI or CT

MANAGEMENT
- None for skin abnormalities

SPECIFIC THERAPY
- None

CAVEATS AND PITFALLS
- No CNS work-up indicated unless there are localizing signs of neurologic disease.

JOGGER'S NIPPLES

ALTERNATE DISEASE NAME
- None

HISTORY
- Occurs in women who do not wear bras when running or in men who wear shirts made of hard, synthetic fibers

PHYSICAL EXAMINATION
- Soreness, dryness, erythema, erosions & bleeding of nipples
- Worse in those w/ erect nipples

DIFFERENTIAL DIAGNOSIS
- Contact dermatitis
- Atopic dermatitis
- Xerotic eczema
- Paget's disease of nipple

LABORATORY WORK-UP
- None

MANAGEMENT
- Protective bras in women
- Soft-fiber outer garments, made of materials such as silk
- Protective tape over nipples before running

SPECIFIC THERAPY
- Emollient creams or petrolatum to nipples before exercise

CAVEATS AND PITFALLS
- None

JUVENILE XANTHOGRANULOMA

ALTERNATE DISEASE NAME
- Nevoxanthoendothelioma
- Xanthoma multiplex
- Juvenile xanthoma
- Congenital xanthoma tuberosum
- Xanthoma naviforme
- Juvenile giant cell granuloma

HISTORY
- Usually occurs in infancy or early childhood in otherwise healthy children
- Occasionally associated w/ eye lesions

PHYSICAL EXAMINATION
- Asymptomatic, smooth, firm papules that initially are red-brown, then change to yellow

- Usually on trunk or upper extremities
- Lesions resolve spontaneously in months to years, leaving small, atrophic scars

DIFFERENTIAL DIAGNOSIS
- Xanthoma
- Mastocytoma
- Insect bite reaction
- Granuloma annulare
- Sarcoidosis
- Spitz nevus
- Langerhans cell histiocytosis
- Non–Langerhans cell histiocytosis
- Benign cephalic histiocytosis
- Generalized eruptive histiocytoma
- Self-healing reticulohistiocytoma
- Xanthoma disseminatum

LABORATORY WORK-UP
- Lesional biopsy if diagnosis is in doubt

MANAGEMENT
- Elliptical excision

SPECIFIC THERAPY
- See "Management"

CAVEATS AND PITFALLS
- Surgical removal for cosmetic reasons only.

KAPOSI'S SARCOMA

ALTERNATE DISEASE NAME
- Kaposi sarcoma
- Multiple idiopathic hemorrhagic sarcoma

HISTORY
- Classic subtype typically affects older men of Mediterranean or eastern European background
- African endemic subtype primarily affects boys & men

- Iatrogenic subtype is seen in kidney & liver transplant pts on immunosuppressive drugs
- AIDS-related subtype occurs in gay men w/ HIV disease

PHYSICAL EXAMINATION
- Classic subtype
  - ➤ May arise in chronically edematous extremities
  - ➤ Violaceous patches, plaques or nodules on lower extremities, which can be painful & can ulcerate
- African endemic subtype
  - ➤ Appears same as classic subtype or in a more deadly form involving bones & lymph system
- Iatrogenic subtype
  - ➤ Appears same as classic subtype
  - ➤ Usually resolves after immunosuppressive drug stopped
- AIDS-related subtype
  - ➤ Lesions often appear on upper body, including oral cavity, head, neck, back & in viscera
  - ➤ Begin as discrete, red or purple patches that are bilaterally symmetric & initially involve lower extremities
  - ➤ Patches become elevated, evolving into nodules & plaques.
  - ➤ May also appear as a large infiltrating mass or as multiple, cone-shaped, friable nodules

DIFFERENTIAL DIAGNOSIS
- Pyogenic granuloma
- Tufted angioma
- Melanocytic nevus
- Melanoma
- Angiokeratoma
- Cavernous hemangioma
- Metastasis
- Arteriovenous malformations

LABORATORY WORK-UP
- Skin biopsy
- HIV test if there is suspicion of this disease

MANAGEMENT
- None indicated for indolent skin tumors in elderly pts

- Localized disease: destructive modalities or intralesional chemotherapy for palliation
- Disseminated disease: chemotherapy

SPECIFIC THERAPY
- Localized disease therapy
  - Liquid nitrogen cryotherapy
  - Localized radiation therapy
  - Elliptical surgical excision
  - Laser ablation
  - Intralesional vinblastine chemotherapy
- Disseminated disease
  - Vinblastine 3.5–10 mg IV weekly, or chemotherapy combinations, w/ vinblastine, bleomycin & doxorubicin
- AIDS-associated disease: antiretroviral therapy

CAVEATS AND PITFALLS
- No therapy is a reasonable option in stable disease, particularly in elderly pts.

KAWASAKI DISEASE

ALTERNATE DISEASE NAME
- Mucocutaneous lymph node syndrome
- Kawasaki syndrome
- Acute febrile mucocutaneous lymph node syndrome

HISTORY
- Most cases in Japan, w/ periodic outbreaks
- Most pts are <5 years old

PHYSICAL EXAMINATION
- Prolonged fever
- Polymorphous exanthem
- Swelling & induration of hands & feet, w/ subsequent desquamation
- Nonexudative conjunctival injection
- Hemorrhagic, crusted, fissured lips
- Bright-red tongue
- Nonsuppurative cervical lymphadenopathy

- Myocarditis & pancarditis
- Coronary artery abnormalities
- Arthralgias & arthritis
- Urethritis w/ sterile pyuria
- Aseptic meningitis
- Diarrhea, vomiting, abdominal pain
- Hydrops of gallbladder
- Auditory abnormalities
- Testicular swelling
- Pneumonitis

DIFFERENTIAL DIAGNOSIS
- Viral exanthem
- Erythema multiforme
- Stevens-Johnson syndrome/toxic epidermal necrolysis
- Scarlet fever
- Rubeola
- Staphylococcal scalded skin syndrome
- Leptospirosis
- Rocky Mountain spotted fever
- Acrodynia
- Juvenile rheumatoid arthritis
- Polyarteritis nodosa

LABORATORY WORK-UP
- Echocardiogram

MANAGEMENT
- Intravenous immunoglobulin (IVIg)
- Aspirin

SPECIFIC THERAPY
- Intravenous immunoglobulin (IVIg), 2 g/kg, as a single infusion over 10–12 hours
- Aspirin 80–100 mg/kg per day PO in 4 divided doses until fever has abated for at least 3 days

CAVEATS AND PITFALLS
- Delay in diagnosis is associated w/ increased coronary artery abnormalities.

KELOID

ALTERNATE DISEASE NAME
- Cheloid
- Keloidal scar

HISTORY
- Familial tendency to develop lesions, w/ or w/out antecedent trauma
- Lesions usually are asymptomatic but may be painful or pruritic
- No spontaneous regression, but may become less discolored over time

PHYSICAL EXAMINATION
- Rubbery or hard, reddish-brown papule or nodule, w/ regular margins, most commonly over earlobes, face, neck, lower extremities, breast, chest, back & abdomen
- May have clawlike projections extending beyond areas of trauma

DIFFERENTIAL DIAGNOSIS
- Hypertrophic scar
- Squamous cell carcinoma
- Dermatofibroma
- Dermatofibrosarcoma protuberans
- Fibromatosis

LABORATORY WORK-UP
- None

MANAGEMENT
- Intralesional corticosteroids
- Cryotherapy
- Silicone gel sheets
- Compression dressings
- Radiation
- Surgical excision w/ postoperative imiquimod or interferon therapy

SPECIFIC THERAPY
- Triamcinolone 10–20 mg/mL intralesional; repeat every 6–8 weeks as needed

CAVEATS AND PITFALLS

- Surgical manipulation or other minor trauma can cause increased growth beyond the original boundaries of the lesion.

KERATOACANTHOMA

ALTERNATE DISEASE NAME

- Self-healing squamous cell carcinoma
- Self-healing epithelioma

HISTORY

- Rapidly enlarging lesion, often on chronically sun-exposed skin
- Rare familial clustering of pts w/multiple lesions

PHYSICAL EXAMINATION

- Solitary, firm, round, skin-colored or reddish papule rapidly progressing to dome-shaped nodule, w/ a smooth shiny surface & a central keratinous plug
- Spontaneous involution possible after many months

DIFFERENTIAL DIAGNOSIS

- Squamous cell carcinoma
- Basal cell carcinoma
- Wart
- Seborrheic keratosis
- Prurigo nodularis
- Inverted follicular keratosis
- Atypical fibroxanthoma
- Merkel cell carcinoma
- Metastasis
- Sporotrichosis
- Coccidioidomycosis
- North American blastomycosis

LABORATORY WORK-UP

- Lesional biopsy, attempting to remove the whole lesion as a single sample

MANAGEMENT

- Surgical excision or destruction

- Radiation therapy
- Intralesional chemotherapy

SPECIFIC THERAPY
- Surgical excision
- Destruction by electrodesiccation & curettage
- Radiation therapy
- Methotrexate 25 mg/mL intralesional, repeated every 2–3 weeks for up to 5 treatments
- Fluorouracil 50 mg/mL intralesional, repeated every 2–3 weeks for up to 5 treatments

CAVEATS AND PITFALLS
- Incomplete removal is associated w/ recurrence of tumor.
- Rare metastatic spread, particularly in tumors on central face.

KERATOSIS PILARIS

ALTERNATE DISEASE NAME
- Lichen pilaris
- Keratosis suprafollicularis
- Pityriasis pilaris

HISTORY
- Usually asymptomatic lesions, w/ usual onset in childhood
- Worse in dry climates & in winter
- Associated w/ atopic dermatitis & ichthyosis vulgaris

PHYSICAL EXAMINATION
- Multiple acuminate follicular keratotic papules, sometimes w/ surrounding erythema
- Most common locations include lateral arms, thighs & cheeks
- Tends to improve w/ age

DIFFERENTIAL DIAGNOSIS
- Lichen spinulosus
- Folliculitis
- Milia
- Ichthyosis
- Pityriasis rubra pilaris

- Darier disease
- Lichen planus
- Phrynoderma

LABORATORY WORK-UP
- None

MANAGEMENT
- Emollients
- Keratolytic agents
- Topical corticosteroids to reduce perilesional inflammation

SPECIFIC THERAPY
- Lactic acid 12% lotion applied BID
- Glycolic acid 5–15% cream or lotion applied BID

CAVEATS AND PITFALLS
- No cure for this condition; should be managed as almost a normal variant.

KYRLE'S DISEASE

ALTERNATE DISEASE NAME
- Kyrle disease
- Hyperkeratosis follicularis et parafollicularis in cutem penetrans

HISTORY
- Eruption most common in pts w/ either diabetes mellitus or renal failure

PHYSICAL EXAMINATION
- Small, scaly papule that enlarges to form red-brown papule or nodule w/ a central keratin plug
- Some follicular papules, which may coalesce to form larger keratotic plaques

DIFFERENTIAL DIAGNOSIS
- Reactive perforating collagenosis
- Perforating folliculitis
- Elastosis perforans serpiginosa
- Prurigo nodularis

- Scabies
- Keratoacanthoma
- Darier disease
- Keratosis pilaris

LABORATORY WORK-UP
- Biopsy only if diagnosis is in doubt

MANAGEMENT
- Systemic vitamin A or retinoids
- Topical retinoids

SPECIFIC THERAPY
- Vitamin A 100,000 units PO daily for 30 days, repeated after a 1-month rest period
- Isotretinoin 1 mg/kg PO daily for 4–6 months

CAVEATS AND PITFALLS
- Isotretinoin is absolutely contraindicated in women of child-bearing potential w/out effective contraception.

LAMELLAR ICHTHYOSIS

ALTERNATE DISEASE NAME
- Nonbullous congenital ichthyosiform erythroderma
- Ichthyosis sebacea
- Ichthyosis congenita larva
- Keratosis rubra congenita

HISTORY
- Present at birth
- Familial clustering

PHYSICAL EXAMINATION
- Newborn presents w/ tough, film-like membrane that fissures when stretched (collodion membrane)
- Membrane sheds in 10–14 days, leaving generalized redness & scale, ranging from fine & white to thick, dark & plate-like, arranged in a pattern resembling fish skin

- Generalized pattern w/ accentuation in flexural areas such as axilla, groin, antecubital fossa & neck, while sparing mucous membranes
- Scarring alopecia
- Nail dystrophy
- Ectropion; eclabium; conjunctivitis
- Small, deformed ears
- Inflexible digits due to taut skin

DIFFERENTIAL DIAGNOSIS
- X-linked ichthyosis
- Congenital ichthyosiform erythroderma
- Conradi disease
- Netherton syndrome
- Trichothiodystrophy
- Erythrodermic psoriasis
- Generalized seborrheic dermatitis
- Rud syndrome
- Sgren-Larsson syndrome

LABORATORY WORK-UP
- Prenatal diagnosis via amniotic fluid or fetal skin biopsy

MANAGEMENT
- Emollients
- Alpha hydroxy acids
- Systemic retinoids

SPECIFIC THERAPY
- Acitretin 25–75 mg PO QD indefinitely

CAVEATS AND PITFALLS
- Advise about possible hyperostoses, osteopenia & premature epiphyseal closure w/ long-term use of systemic retinoids.

LANGERHANS CELL HISTIOCYTOSIS

ALTERNATE DISEASE NAME
- Histiocytosis X
- Langerhans cell granulomatosis
- Type II histiocytosis

HISTORY
- Unifocal disease is often asymptomatic
- Disseminated disease may present w/ signs & symptoms suggestive of acute infection or malignancy

PHYSICAL EXAMINATION
- Unifocal disease (eosinophilic granuloma): solitary bony lesion, which is usually asymptomatic
- Multifocal disease (Hand-Schuler-Christian variant)
  - Diabetes insipidus, bony defects & exophthalmos
  - Other systemic features include liver, spleen, lymph node infiltration
  - Skin lesions include noduloulcerative lesions in oral, perineal, perivulvar or retroauricular regions
- Acute disseminated disease (Letterer-Siwe variant)
  - Skin findings include petechiae; scaly or crusted yellow-brown papules, sometimes coalescing to form plaques, often in seborrheic distribution, & exudative intertriginous lesions, which may ulcerate
  - Systemic findings include fever, anemia, thrombocytopenia, pulmonary infiltrates, enlargement of lymph nodes, spleen & liver & neurologic involvement

DIFFERENTIAL DIAGNOSIS
- Seborrheic dermatitis
- Candidiasis
- Herpes simplex virus infection
- Varicella
- Dermatomyositis
- Mastocytosis
- Wiskott-Aldrich syndrome
- Acrodermatitis enteropathica
- Rosai-Dorfman disease
- Xanthoma disseminatum
- Listeriosis
- Infantile acropustulosis
- Leukemia
- Lymphoma
- Myeloma

LABORATORY WORK-UP
- CBC & differential
- Reticulocyte count
- Erythrocyte sedimentation rate
- Direct & indirect Coombs test
- Immunoglobulin levels
- Bone radiographs as indicated by clinical exam
- CT scan or MRI of hypothalamic-pituitary region if indicated by clinical exam

MANAGEMENT
- Localized skin involvement: topical corticosteroids
- Extensive skin involvement
  - Topical nitrogen mustard
  - Photochemotherapy
- Multisystem disease: chemotherapy

SPECIFIC THERAPY
- Fluocinonide 0.05% cream applied BID Nitrogen mustard ointment applied QD, using the following recipe:
  - Mechlorethamine hydrochloride
    - 90 mg
  - Absolute alcohol (ethyl or isopropyl)
    - 10 mL
  - Aquaphor Ointment
    - 900 g

CAVEATS AND PITFALLS
- Unclear whether aggressive therapy prolongs survival in advanced disease.

LARGE PLAQUE PARAPSORIASIS

ALTERNATE DISEASE NAME
- Interface parapsoriasis
- Atrophic parapsoriasis
- Variegate dermatitis

HISTORY
- Begins as a few patches & becomes more visible over a long period of time

PHYSICAL EXAMINATION
- Faint, salmon-colored plaques w/ arcuate geographic borders, often >5 cm in diameter
- May have an atrophic or tissue-paper surface quality
- Lesions occur on proximal extremities & trunk in a bathing trunk distribution
- Rare spontaneous remission
- May progress to cutaneous T-cell lymphoma after many years

DIFFERENTIAL DIAGNOSIS
- Small plaque parapsoriasis
- Psoriasis
- Mycosis fungoides
- Seborrheic dermatitis
- Dermatophytosis
- Lupus erythematosus
- Lichen planus
- Pityriasis rosea
- Syphilis
- Xerosis
- Nummular dermatitis

LABORATORY WORK-UP
- Skin biopsy

MANAGEMENT
- Phototherapy
- Topical corticosteroids

SPECIFIC THERAPY
- Fluocinonide 0.05 w% cream applied BID

CAVEATS AND PITFALLS
- Only minor response to topical therapy.

LEISHMANIASIS, CUTANEOUS

ALTERNATE DISEASE NAME
- Aleppo boil
- Delhi boil

- Bagdad boil
- Biskra button
- Oriental sore

HISTORY
- Endemic in Middle East, Central & South America
- Occurs several weeks to months (rarely years) after sandfly bite inoculation on exposed skin

PHYSICAL EXAMINATION
- Asymptomatic red papule that ulcerates, at site of sandfly bite
- Spontaneous healing after weeks to many months

DIFFERENTIAL DIAGNOSIS
- Cutaneous tuberculosis
- Deep fungal infection
- Pyoderma gangrenosum
- Syphilis
- Leprosy
- Basal cell carcinoma
- Squamous cell carcinoma

LABORATORY WORK-UP
- Skin biopsy for light microscopy & tissue culture

MANAGEMENT
- Pentavalent antimony
- Ketoconazole
- Amphotericin B
- Localized hyperthermia

SPECIFIC THERAPY
- Sodium antimony gluconate 20 mg/kg per day IV or IM for 20 days
- Ketoconazole 600 mg PO daily for 4 weeks
- Amphotericin B (w/ deoxycholate): 1 mg/kg IV for 20 days

CAVEATS AND PITFALLS
- Lesions may appear asynchronously over several weeks after single exposure.

LENTIGO

ALTERNATE DISEASE NAME
- Sun spot
- Liver spot

HISTORY
- Gradual onset of asymptomatic brown spots

PHYSICAL EXAMINATION
- Lentigo simplex
  - ➤ Round or oval, uniformly tan-brown to black macules, w/ jagged or smooth margins
  - ➤ Lesions few in number & occur anywhere on skin or mucous membranes
- Solar lentigo
  - ➤ Occurs most commonly on face, arms, dorsa of hands & upper part of trunk
  - ➤ Stellate-shaped, round or oval, uniformly tan-brown to black macules; slowly increasing in number & in size
  - ➤ Macules may coalesce to form larger patches
- Ink spot lentigo
  - ➤ Reticulated pattern, resembling spot of ink; limited to sun-exposed areas
  - ➤ Most common presentation is a single lesion among many solar lentigines
- Tanning-bed lentigo
  - ➤ Usually appears in women w/ history of tanning-bed use
  - ➤ Similar in appearance to PUVA lentigo
- PUVA lentigo
  - ➤ Occurrence associated w/ greater cumulative doses of PUVA
  - ➤ Persistent, pale brown macule appearing 6 months or longer after start of PUVA therapy
  - ➤ Resembles solar lentigo, but often w/ more irregular borders, which may mimic ephelides
- Radiation lentigo
  - ➤ Similar in appearance to solar lentigo, but has other histopathologic signs of long-term cutaneous radiation damage

- Mucosal melanotic macule
  - ➤ Labial lentigo: almost always occurs as solitary pigmented macule on vermilion of lower lip
  - ➤ Oral lentigo: appears on gingiva, buccal mucosa, palate & tongue
  - ➤ Penile lentigo: most common sites include glans penis, corona, corona sulcus & penile shaft
  - ➤ Vulvar lentigo: appears anywhere on the genital mucosa as a mottled, pigmented patch w/ skip areas

DIFFERENTIAL DIAGNOSIS
- Melanocytic nevus
- Lentigo maligna
- Melanoma
- Ephelides
- Actinic keratosis
- Seborrheic keratosis
- Traumatic tattoo
- Phytophotodermatitis

LABORATORY WORK-UP
- Skin biopsy if there is concern about possible melanoma

MANAGEMENT
- Therapy for cosmetic reasons only
- Laser ablation w/ frequency-doubled Q-switched Nd:YAG laser, or HGM K1 krypton laser or 532-nm diode-pumped vanadate laser
- Bleaching agents

SPECIFIC THERAPY
- Hydroquinone 4% cream, w/ or w/out tretinoin, applied QD for at least 3 months

CAVEATS AND PITFALLS
- Often incomplete response to bleaching agent treatment.

LEPROSY

ALTERNATE DISEASE NAME
- Hansen's disease
- Hansen disease

HISTORY
- Severity & extent of disease depend on genetic susceptibility
- Minimal prodrome

PHYSICAL EXAMINATION
- Indeterminate leprosy: one to a few hypopigmented or erythematous macules, w/ intact sensation
- Tuberculoid leprosy
  - Skin lesions few in number; well-defined, erythematous large plaques, w/ elevated borders that slope down into an atrophic center
  - Lesions found on face, limbs or elsewhere, but sparing intertriginous areas & scalp
  - Alternate presentation: large, asymmetric, hypopigmented macule
  - Both types of lesions are anesthetic, involving alopecia & sometimes spontaneously resolving in a few years, leaving pigmentary disturbances or scars
  - Neural involvement leading to tender, thickened nerves w/ subsequent loss of function
  - Great auricular nerve & superficial peroneal nerves often prominent
- Borderline tuberculoid leprosy: similar to tuberculoid form, but lesions smaller & more numerous, nerves less enlarged & less alopecia
- Borderline leprosy
  - Numerous, asymmetric, moderately anesthetic, red, irregularly shaped plaques, which are less well defined than those in tuberculoid type
  - Regional adenopathy may be present
- Lepromatous leprosy: only infectious stage
  - Early cutaneous lesions consisting mainly of pale, small, diffuse, symmetric macules, which become infiltrated later, w/ little loss of sensation
  - Nerves not thickened & sweating normal
  - Alopecia of lateral eyebrows, eyelashes & then trunk, but scalp hair remains normal
  - Diffuse nodules (lepromas) or plaques, which result in appearance of leonine facies

- ➤ Brawny lower extremity edema
- ➤ Neuritic lesions symmetric & slow to develop
- ➤ Eye involvement causing pain, photophobia, decreased visual acuity, glaucoma, blindness
- ➤ Testicular atrophy leading to sterility & gynecomastia
- ➤ Lymphadenopathy & hepatomegaly from organ infiltration
- ➤ Stridor & hoarseness from laryngeal involvement
- ➤ Nasal infiltration sometimes causing a saddle-nose deformity; aseptic necrosis & osteomyelitis
- ■ Reactional state
  - ➤ Lepra type I reaction
    - • Usually affects pts w/ borderline disease
    - • Downgrading reaction is shift toward lepromatous pole before initiation of therapy
    - • Reversal reaction is shifting of disease toward tuberculoid pole after initiation of therapy
  - ➤ Lepra type II reactions (erythema nodosum leprosum)
    - • Immune complex-mediated reaction occurring in pts w/ borderline lepromatous or polar lepromatous disease
    - • Crops of painful red papules, usually occurring after a few years of therapy & resolving spontaneously after about 5 years
    - • Associated fever, malaise, joint pain, nerve pain, iridocyclitis, dactylitis & orchitis
- ■ Lucio phenomenon
  - ➤ Common in Mexico & Central America
  - ➤ Cutaneous hemorrhagic infarcts in pts w/ diffuse lepromatous disease

DIFFERENTIAL DIAGNOSIS
- ■ Vitiligo
- ■ Postinflammatory hypopigmentation
- ■ Lupus erythematosus
- ■ Tuberculosis
- ■ Syphilis
- ■ Sarcoidosis
- ■ Leishmaniasis
- ■ Granuloma annulare
- ■ Psoriasis

LABORATORY WORK-UP
- Skin biopsy
- Tissue smear testing, where an incision is made in the skin & the blade is used to obtain tissue fluid for examination w/ Ziehl-Nielson stain

MANAGEMENT
- Multidrug antibiotic therapy
- Reactional states
  - Systemic corticosteroids
  - Thalidomide

SPECIFIC THERAPY
- Paucibacillary disease
  - Dapsone 100 mg PO QD; titrate as per response
  - Rifampin 300 mg PO BID for 3 months
- Multibacillary disease
  - Dapsone 100 mg PO QD indefinitely
  - Rifampin 300 mg PO BID for 3 years
  - Clofazimine 50 mg PO per day for 3 years
- Reactional states
  - Prednisone 0.5–2 mg/kg PO QAM until reaction subsides
  - Thalidomide 100–300 mg PO QD

CAVEATS AND PITFALLS
- If prednisone is to be used for >21 days per course of therapy, obtain baseline chest radiograph, TB skin test & bone mineral density determination.
- If thalidomide is used, advise about possible peripheral neuropathy & absolute contraindication w/ pregnancy.
- Check CBC Q2–3 weeks for 10–12 weeks w/ dapsone to detect rare pancytopenia.
- Obtain baseline G6PD level before dapsone therapy.

LEPTOSPIROSIS

ALTERNATE DISEASE NAME
- Autumnal fever
- 7-day fever

- Seven-day fever
- Canefield fever
- Swineherd's disease
- Swamp fever
- Mud fever
- Fort Bragg fever
- Weil disease

HISTORY
- Sources of direct infection include body fluids or organs of infected animals
- Sources of indirect infection include inoculated soil or water

PHYSICAL EXAMINATION
- Anicteric leptospirosis: self-limited disease similar to a mild flu-like illness
- Icteric leptospirosis
  - Severe illness characterized by multiple organ system involvement; skin changes: warm & flushed
  - Transient petechial eruption that can involve the palate
  - Jaundice & purpura w/ severe disease
  - Conjunctival suffusion
  - Myalgia
  - Signs of meningitis, including neck stiffness & rigidity, delirium, photophobia
  - Hepatomegaly & tenderness from hepatitis

DIFFERENTIAL DIAGNOSIS
- Enteric fever
- Viral hepatitis
- Hantavirus infection
- Rickettsial disease
- Encephalitis
- Typhoid fever
- Dengue fever
- Viral meningitis
- Malaria

LABORATORY WORK-UP
- Skin biopsy for histologic evaluation & culture
- Urine, blood cultures

MANAGEMENT
- Systemic antibiotics

SPECIFIC THERAPY
- Mild disease
  - ➤ Doxycycline 100 mg PO BID for 21 days
  - ➤ Amoxicillin 0.5–1 g PO TID for 14–21 days
  - ➤ Erythromycin 250–500 mg QID for 21 days
- Severe disease
  - ➤ Penicillin G 20–24 million units IV per day, divided into 4 doses for 5–10 days

CAVEATS AND PITFALLS
- None

LEUKOCYTOCLASTIC VASCULITIS

ALTERNATE DISEASE NAME
- Allergic cutaneous vasculitis
- Allergic angiitis
- Small vessel vasculitis

HISTORY
- May occur in the absence of any systemic disease
- May appear in conjunction w/ rheumatic disorders, paraproteinemia, ingestants (drugs or foods), infections or malignancy

PHYSICAL EXAMINATION
- Asymptomatic, pruritic or painful, palpable purpuric or urticarial papules, sometimes coalescing into plaques and/or ulcerating
- Occurs most frequently on legs, but any surface possible
- Systemic manifestations of lung, GI, renal or rheumatologic involvement reflected in signs & symptoms referable to those organs

DIFFERENTIAL DIAGNOSIS
- Septic vasculitis (eg, meningococcemia, gonococcemia)
- Benign pigmented purpura
- Wegener granulomatosis

- Polyarteritis nodosa
- Erythema multiforme
- Infective endocarditis
- Churg-Strauss syndrome
- Cholesterol emboli
- Amyloidosis
- Buerger disease
- Rocky Mountain spotted fever
- Thrombotic thrombocytopenic purpura
- Urticaria
- Waldenström hypergammaglobulinemia
- Idiopathic thrombocytopenia purpura or other causes of decreased platelets

LABORATORY WORK-UP
- Skin biopsy
- CBC, ESR, urinalysis, blood chemistry panel
- Serologic tests, complement level, cryoglobulin if rheumatic disease suspected

MANAGEMENT
- Severe, recalcitrant disease
  - ➤ Systemic corticosteroids
  - ➤ Colchicine

SPECIFIC THERAPY
- Prednisone 1 mg/kg PO QAM for up to 3 weeks
- Colchicine 0.6–1.8 mg PO QD

CAVEATS AND PITFALLS
- No therapy indicated for mild, asymptomatic disease.
- Consider steroid-sparing drugs if prednisone is to be used for >3 weeks.
- Advise about diarrhea as dose-limiting side effect of colchicine.

LICHEN AMYLOIDOSIS

ALTERNATE DISEASE NAME
- Primary localized cutaneous amyloidosis

HISTORY
- Intense pruritus precedes the eruption in many cases
- Not associated w/ systemic amyloidosis

PHYSICAL EXAMINATION
- Intensely pruritic, flesh-colored or red-brown, hyperkeratotic papules, most commonly seen on pretibial surfaces but also on feet & thighs
- Macular variant: irregular hyperpigmented patches over back or chest, which may not be as pruritic as lichen amyloid variant

DIFFERENTIAL DIAGNOSIS
- Postinflammatory hyperpigmentation
- Lichen simplex chronicus
- Prurigo nodularis
- Ashy dermatosis
- Mycosis fungoides
- Contact dermatitis
- Lichen planus
- Lichenoid drug eruption
- Pretibial myxedema
- Necrobiosis lipoidica
- Acanthosis nigricans

LABORATORY WORK-UP
- Skin biopsy for routine histology, w/ amyloid stains

MANAGEMENT
- Topical corticosteroids for associated eczema
- Cyclosporine for severe disease associated w/ atopic dermatitis

SPECIFIC THERAPY
- Clobetasol 0.05 w% cream applied BID
- Cyclosporine 3–5 mg/kg PO QD for up to 6 months

CAVEATS AND PITFALLS
- Topical corticosteroid therapy has little effect on amyloid deposits.
- Monitor renal function & blood pressure w/ cyclosporine therapy.

LICHEN NITIDUS

ALTERNATE DISEASE NAME
- None

HISTORY
- Insidious onset of asymptomatic eruption

PHYSICAL EXAMINATION
- Multiple 1- to 3-mm, sharply demarcated, clustered, round or polygonal, flat-topped, skin-colored shiny papules
- Occur most commonly on trunk, thighs, forearms, genitalia
- Köebner phenomenon may occur

DIFFERENTIAL DIAGNOSIS
- Flat warts
- Lichen spinulosus
- Lichen amyloidosis
- Keratosis pilaris
- Lichen striatus
- Lichen planus
- Id reaction
- Sarcoidosis

LABORATORY WORK-UP
- None

MANAGEMENT
- Topical corticosteroids

SPECIFIC THERAPY
- Fluocinonide 0.05% cream applied BID

CAVEATS AND PITFALLS
- None

LICHEN PLANUS

ALTERNATE DISEASE NAME
- Lichen rubor

HISTORY
- Insidious or sudden onset of pruritic eruption
- Oral lesions may be asymptomatic unless there are erosions

PHYSICAL EXAMINATION

- Pruritic, discrete or confluent, polygonal violaceous papules, w/ fine white scale (Wickham's stria)
- Mucous membrane involvement w/ white or gray streaks forming a linear or reticular pattern on a violaceous background, most commonly on buccal mucosa & tongue
- Genital involvement w/ annular papules on glans penis
- Vulvar involvement w/ reticulate papules or erosions, w/ dyspareunia, burning sensation, pruritus & vulvar & urethral stenosis
- Nail plate thinning w/ longitudinal grooving & ridging & occasional destruction of nail plate w/ pterygium formation
- Follicular & perifollicular, violaceous, scaly, pruritic papules on scalp, sometimes progressing to atrophic cicatricial alopecia (lichen planopilaris)
- Hypertrophic variant: pruritic, thick, scaly, violaceous plaques, usually on anterior leg
- Atrophic variant: few lesions, often representing resolution of annular or hypertrophic lesions
- Erosive variant: chronic, painful erosions on mucosal surfaces, which evolve from sites of previous nonerosive disease
- Actinic variant: nummular plaques w/ a hypopigmented zone surrounding a hyperpigmented center

DIFFERENTIAL DIAGNOSIS

- Lichenoid drug eruption
- Psoriasis
- Pityriasis rosea
- Lupus erythematosus
- Scabies
- Chronic graft-versus-host disease
- Lichen simplex chronicus
- Lichen nitidus
- Syphilis
- Pemphigus foliaceus
- Squamous cell carcinoma of oral mucosa

LABORATORY WORK-UP

- Skin biopsy only if diagnosis is in doubt

MANAGEMENT
- Localized disease: topical corticosteroids
- Extensive disease
  - Systemic corticosteroids
  - Photochemotherapy
  - Systemic retinoids

SPECIFIC THERAPY
- Clobetasol 0.05% cream applied BID
- Prednisone 1 mg/kg PO QAM for up to 3 weeks
- Acitretin 25–75 mg PO QD
- Isotretinoin 1 mg/kg PO QD for up to 6 months

CAVEATS AND PITFALLS
- Systemic retinoids are contraindicated in pregnancy.

LICHEN SCLEROSUS

ALTERNATE DISEASE NAME
- Lichen sclerosus et atrophicus
- Kraurosis vulvae
- Balanitis xerotica obliterans

HISTORY
- Vulvar disease usually presents w/ progressive pruritus, dyspareunia, dysuria or genital bleeding
- Penile disease usually starts w/ pruritus but may present w/ sudden phimosis of previously retractable foreskin
- Extragenital disease is usually asymptomatic

PHYSICAL EXAMINATION
- White, polygonal papules coalescing into shiny plaques, often w/ follicular prominence & occasional isomorphic response (Köebner phenomenon)
- Vulvar variant (kraurosis vulvae)
  - Gradual obliteration of labia minora & stenosis of introitus
  - Occasional blisters or hemorrhagic bullae
  - Hourglass pattern involving perivaginal & perianal areas

- Male genital variant (balanitis xerotica obliterans)
  - Usually confined to glans penis & prepuce or foreskin remnants
  - May produce phimosis after extensive sclerosis of prepuce

DIFFERENTIAL DIAGNOSIS
- Morphea or other forms of scleroderma
- Idiopathic guttate hypomelanosis
- Child abuse
- Lichen planus
- Psoriasis
- Tinea versicolor
- Vitiligo
- Postinflammatory hypopigmentation
- Anetoderma
- Bowen's disease

LABORATORY WORK-UP
- Skin biopsy if diagnosis is in doubt

MANAGEMENT
- Genital disease
  - Topical corticosteroids
  - Systemic retinoids

SPECIFIC THERAPY
- Clobetasol 0.05% cream applied BID
- Acitretin 25–50 mg PO QD
- Isotretinoin 1 mg/kg PO QD for 4–6 months

CAVEATS AND PITFALLS
- Systemic retinoids are contraindicated in pregnancy.
- No effective therapy for extragenital disease.

LICHEN SIMPLEX CHRONICUS

ALTERNATE DISEASE NAME
- Neurodermatitis circumscripta
- Circumscribed neurodermatitis
- Lichen simplex chronicus of Vidal

HISTORY

- Paroxysmal pruritus in localized area, almost always at site that is easily reached for scratching

PHYSICAL EXAMINATION

- One or more slightly erythematous, scaly, well-demarcated, lichenified, firm plaques, often w/ hyperpigmentation
- Most common sites of involvement include posterior neck, scalp, extensor aspect of extremities, vulva in women & scrotum in men
- Prurigo nodularis variant
  - Discrete, firm, purpuric nodules or papules, often w/ overlying erosion
  - Occurs on extensor surfaces of arms & legs, posterior neck, upper back & trunk

DIFFERENTIAL DIAGNOSIS

- Atopic dermatitis
- Acanthosis nigricans
- Nummular eczema
- Contact dermatitis
- Stasis dermatitis
- Lichen amyloidosis
- Insect bite reaction
- Psoriasis
- Lupus erythematosus
- Dermatophytosis
- Lichen planus
- Acne keloidalis

LABORATORY WORK-UP

- None

MANAGEMENT

- Topical and/or intralesional corticosteroids
- Systemic antihistamines, used as sedatives

SPECIFIC THERAPY

- Triamcinolone 0.1% cream applied BID
- Flurandrenolide tape, applied continuously for 2 weeks
- Triamcinolone 3–4 mg/mL intralesional; repeat in 6 weeks prn

CAVEATS AND PITFALLS
- Flurandrenolide tape can produce severe skin atrophy if used for >2 weeks w/out a 1-week rest period between courses.

LICHEN SPINULOSUS

ALTERNATE DISEASE NAME
- Keratosis follicularis spinulosa
- Lichen pilaris spinulosus of Crocker
- Keratosis follicularis spinosa of Unna

HISTORY
- Sudden onset of asymptomatic lesions

PHYSICAL EXAMINATION
- Plaques consisting of acuminate, keratotic papules
- Occurs on neck, buttocks, abdomen, trochanters, knees & extensor surfaces of arms

DIFFERENTIAL DIAGNOSIS
- Lichen nitidus
- Keratosis pilaris
- Lichen simplex chronicus
- Flat warts
- Phrynoderma
- Lichen planopilaris
- Pityriasis rubra pilaris
- Darier disease

LABORATORY WORK-UP
- None

MANAGEMENT
- Keratolytic agents

SPECIFIC THERAPY
- Lactic acid 12% lotion applied BID
- Urea 20–40% cream applied BID

CAVEATS AND PITFALLS
- Only minimal benefit from keratolytic agents.

LICHEN STRIATUS

ALTERNATE DISEASE NAME
- Linear eczema
- Linear lichenoid dermatosis
- Linear neurodermatitis
- Blaschkitis
- Blaschko linear acquired inflammatory skin eruption
- Zonal dermatosis
- Linear dermatosis

HISTORY
- Sudden onset of asymptomatic localized eruption, usually on an extremity or trunk
- Progresses from proximal to distal

PHYSICAL EXAMINATION
- Flat-topped, erythematous or skin-colored, lichenoid, scaly papules, coalescing into small plaques in a continuous or interrupted linear band
- Spontaneous resolution in months to 1 year, often in the same proximal-to-distal fashion in which they appeared, leaving variable dyspigmentation

DIFFERENTIAL DIAGNOSIS
- Inflammatory linear verrucous epidermal nevus
- Lichen simplex chronicus
- Wart
- Lichen planus
- Atopic dermatitis
- Darier disease
- Porokeratosis

LABORATORY WORK-UP
- None

MANAGEMENT
- Topical corticosteroids

SPECIFIC THERAPY
- Fluocinonide 0.05% cream applied BID

CAVEATS AND PITFALLS
- Minimal benefit of topical therapy.

LICHENOID KERATOSIS

ALTERNATE DISEASE NAME
- Benign lichenoid keratosis
- Solitary lichen planus
- Solitary lichen planus-like keratosis
- Lichenoid benign keratosis

HISTORY
- Usually arises from pre-existing lesion, either lentigo or seborrheic keratosis
- Associated w/ variable pruritus and pain

PHYSICAL EXAMINATION
- Sharply demarcated, scaly, red-brown, almost flat papule, often on sun-exposed skin of extremities

DIFFERENTIAL DIAGNOSIS
- Lentigo
- Seborrheic keratosis
- Lichen planus
- Lichenoid drug eruption
- Lupus erythematosus
- Wart
- Bowen's disease
- Superficial basal cell carcinoma

LABORATORY WORK-UP
- Biopsy if diagnosis is in doubt

MANAGEMENT
- Local destructive modality

SPECIFIC THERAPY
- Destruction by electrodesiccation & curettage
- Liquid nitrogen cryotherapy

CAVEATS AND PITFALLS
- None

LINEAR IGA DERMATOSIS

ALTERNATE DISEASE NAME
- Linear IgA bullous dermatosis
- Linear IgA bullous disease
- Chronic bullous disease of childhood

HISTORY
- May have prodromal itching or transient pruritus or burning before lesions appear
- Sudden onset if related to medication, particularly vancomycin; otherwise gradual onset

PHYSICAL EXAMINATION
- Clear and/or hemorrhagic vesicles or bullae on normal, erythematous or urticarial skin
- May have erythematous plaques, blanching macules & papules or erythema multiforme-like lesions
- May have oral mucous membrane lesions, including red patches, vesicles, ulcerations, erosions, desquamative gingivitis or cheilitis

DIFFERENTIAL DIAGNOSIS
- Bullous pemphigoid
- Erythema multiforme
- Dermatitis herpetiformis
- Pemphigus foliaceous
- Epidermolysis bullosa acquisita
- Impetigo
- Pemphigus vulgaris
- Herpes simplex virus infection
- Herpes zoster
- Epidermolysis bullosa

LABORATORY WORK-UP
- Skin biopsy for routine histology & direct immunofluorescence

MANAGEMENT
- Systemic corticosteroids
- Sulfones
- Combination of tetracycline & niacinamide

SPECIFIC THERAPY
- Dapsone 25–100 mg PO QD; titrate as per response after 2 weeks
- Prednisone 1 mg/kg PO QAM
- Tetracycline 500 mg PO 2 or 3 times daily
- Niacinamide 500 mg PO 2 or 3 times daily

CAVEATS AND PITFALLS
- Attempt conservative therapy w/ combination of tetracycline & niacinamide first in early or mild disease.
- If prednisone is to be used for >21 days per course of therapy, obtain baseline chest radiograph, TB skin test & bone mineral density determination.
- Check CBC Q2–3 weeks for 10–12 weeks w/ dapsone to detect rare pancytopenia.
- Obtain baseline G6PD level before dapsone therapy.

LIPOID PROTEINOSIS

ALTERNATE DISEASE NAME
- Hyalinosis cutis et mucosae
- Urbach-Wiethe disease
- Lipoproteinosis
- Lipoglycoproteinosis
- Lipoidosis cutis et mucosae

HISTORY
- Familial clustering
- Hoarse or weak cry in infancy
- Involvement of larynx & vocal cords may cause respiratory distress
- Children may have behavioral or learning difficulties and/or a seizure disorder

PHYSICAL EXAMINATION
- Begins early in life w/ recurrent vesicles, bullae & hemorrhagic crusts, particularly on face, in mucous membranes & distal extremities, which heal w/ ice-pick scarring
- Later in life, skin becomes waxy, thickened & yellow, w/ papules, plaques & nodules on face, axillae & scrotum
- Verrucous lesions on elbows, knees & sites of trauma
- Beaded papules along eyelid margins (moniliform blepharitis)
- Patchy alopecia
- Cobblestone appearance of multiple papules on tongue, lips, gingiva
- Tongue may feel hard, w/ woody induration & ulceration

DIFFERENTIAL DIAGNOSIS
- Amyloidosis
- Papular mucinosis
- Xanthomas
- Colloid milia
- Myxedema
- Erythropoietic protoporphyria

LABORATORY WORK-UP
- Skin biopsy to confirm diagnosis
- CT of head if there are suggestive signs & symptoms

MANAGEMENT
- Systemic retinoids
- Dermabrasion
- Surgical resection of vocal cord papules

SPECIFIC THERAPY
- Acitretin 25–50 mg PO QD for up to 5 months

CAVEATS AND PITFALLS
- Systemic retinoids are contraindicated in women of child-bearing potential.

LIPOMA

ALTERNATE DISEASE NAME
- Fatty tumor
- Lipomatosis

HISTORY
- Insidious onset of slow-growing, asymptomatic soft tissue growth

PHYSICAL EXAMINATION
- Soft, subcutaneous nodule, most commonly over back, neck, shoulders & proximal upper extremities

DIFFERENTIAL DIAGNOSIS
- Epidermoid cyst
- Liposarcoma
- Neurofibroma
- Panniculitis
- Leiomyoma
- Blue rubber bleb nevus syndrome
- Glomus tumor

LABORATORY WORK-UP
- Lesional biopsy only if diagnosis is in doubt

MANAGEMENT
- Surgical excision
- Liposuction

SPECIFIC THERAPY
- See "Management"

CAVEATS AND PITFALLS
- None

LIVEDOID VASCULITIS

ALTERNATE DISEASE NAME
- Livedo vasculitis
- Livedo reticularis w/ summer/winter ulcerations
- Segmental hyalinizing vasculitis

HISTORY
- More frequent in women, w/ seasonal flares in summer & winter
- May have a history of livedo reticularis of lower legs
- May have associated blood factor deficiencies

PHYSICAL EXAMINATION
- Starts as small, painful, purpuric macules & papules that ulcerate & heal w/ stellate white atrophic scars, w/ surrounding telangiectasias & hyperpigmentation

DIFFERENTIAL DIAGNOSIS
- Livedo reticularis (retiform purpura)
- Hypersensitivity vasculitis
- Stasis ulceration
- Cholesterol emboli
- Septic emboli
- Antiphospholipid antibody syndrome
- Lupus erythematosus

LABORATORY WORK-UP
- Lesional biopsy

MANAGEMENT
- Antiplatelet therapy
- Fibrinolytic agents
- Anticoagulants
- Pentoxifylline

SPECIFIC THERAPY
- Aspirin 325 mg PO QD & dipyridamole 75 mg PO QID
- Danazol 200 mg PO QD
- Enoxaparin 1 mg/kg q12h
- Pentoxifylline 400 mg PO TID

CAVEATS AND PITFALLS
- May be final common pathway of several different disorders.

LUPUS ERYTHEMATOSUS, ACUTE

ALTERNATE DISEASE NAME
- Acute lupus erythematosus

HISTORY
- Rapid onset of signs & symptoms, including skin eruption
- May occur shortly after excess sun exposure

PHYSICAL EXAMINATION
- Confluent erythema & edema, most commonly over malar eminence & nasal bridge (butterfly eruption)
- Vesicles & bullae, often over lower extremities
- Morbilliform macules & papules in a sunlight distribution & forehead, periorbital area & sides of neck
- Superficial ulceration, primarily involving posterior surface of hard palate

DIFFERENTIAL DIAGNOSIS
- Rosacea
- Tinea faciei
- Seborrheic dermatitis
- Dermatomyositis
- Polymorphous light eruption
- Erythema multiforme
- Phototoxic drug eruption
- Solar urticaria

LABORATORY WORK-UP
- Rheumatic disease serologies, including ANA, anti-Sm, RO/SSA, anti-native DNA antibodies
- Serum complement
- Serum chemistries, including CBC, renal function studies
- Skin biopsy for routine histology

MANAGEMENT
- Systemic corticosteroids
- Steroid-sparing agents
- IVIG

SPECIFIC THERAPY
- Prednisone 0.5–1 mg/kg PO QAM
- Steroid-sparing agents
  - Azathioprine 2–3 mg/kg PO QD
  - Cyclophosphamide 50–200 mg PO QD or as monthly pulse therapy
  - Thalidomide 100–300 mg PO QD
  - Hydroxychloroquine 200 mg PO BID
- IVIG: 0.5–1 g/kg per day for 4 days

CAVEATS AND PITFALLS
- If prednisone is to be used for >21 days per course of therapy, obtain baseline chest radiograph, TB skin test & bone mineral density determination.
- Check thiopurine methyltransferase levels before starting azathioprine therapy.
- Check for possible retinal toxicity w/ hydroxychloroquine every 6 months.

LUPUS ERYTHEMATOSUS, CHRONIC CUTANEOUS

ALTERNATE DISEASE NAME
- Chronic cutaneous lupus erythematosus
- Discoid lupus erythematosus

HISTORY
- Gradual onset of asymptomatic or mildly pruritic skin lesions, usually w/out any other signs or symptoms of systemic disease
- Sun exposure is antecedent event in some cases.

PHYSICAL EXAMINATION
- Minimally scaly, erythematous papule or plaque, evolving w/ hypopigmentation in central area & hyperpigmentation at active border
- As lesion evolves, dilation of follicular openings occurs w/ keratinous plug (follicular plugging; patulous follicles).
- Resolution results in atrophy & scarring.
- Localized variant: occurs when only head & neck affected, w/ few lesions
- Widespread variant
  - Occurs when areas other than head & neck affected, often w/ multiple lesions
  - More likely to develop systemic lupus erythematosus

DIFFERENTIAL DIAGNOSIS
- Lichen planus
- Actinic keratosis
- Granuloma faciale
- Jessner lymphocytic infiltration of skin

- Granuloma annulare
- Sarcoidosis
- Dermatomyositis
- Rosacea
- Tinea faciei
- Squamous cell carcinoma

LABORATORY WORK-UP
- Skin biopsy
- Serum chemistries, looking for evidence of organ dysfunction, particularly kidney, liver & bone marrow

MANAGEMENT
- Topical corticosteroids
- Intralesional corticosteroids
- Antimalarials

SPECIFIC THERAPY
- Clobetasol 0.05% cream applied BID
- Triamcinolone 3–4 mg/mL intralesional; repeat in 6 weeks prn
- Hydroxychloroquine 200 mg PO BID
- Prednisone 0.5–1 mg/kg PO QAM; use only if hydroxychloroquine fails

CAVEATS AND PITFALLS
- Check for possible retinal toxicity w/ hydroxychloroquine every 6 months.
- Use prednisone only after hydroxychloroquine failure.
- If prednisone is to be used for >21 days per course of therapy, obtain baseline chest radiograph, TB skin test & bone mineral density determination.

LUPUS ERYTHEMATOSUS, SUBACUTE

ALTERNATE DISEASE NAME
- Subacute cutaneous lupus erythematosus

HISTORY
- Several drugs may produce this syndrome, most commonly thiazide diuretics.

■ May be manifestation of systemic lupus erythematosus or have no associated internal manifestations

PHYSICAL EXAMINATION
■ Starts as a minimally scaly, erythematous papule or a small plaque, usually in sun-exposed distribution
■ Associated systemic signs & symptoms include Sjgren syndrome, fatigue, arthritis, pleuritis & pericarditis.
■ Papulosquamous variant: may mimic psoriasis or lichen planus
■ Annular variant: similar to erythema annulare centrifugum
■ Neonatal type
  ➤ Transient infiltrated red papules & plaques on face
  ➤ Lesions usually resolve by age 4–6 months
  ➤ Some pts develop heart block, requiring pacemaker.

DIFFERENTIAL DIAGNOSIS
■ Psoriasis
■ Erythema annulare centrifugum
■ Polymorphous light eruption
■ Erythema multiforme
■ Tinea corporis
■ Lichen planus
■ Sarcoidosis
■ Granuloma annulare
■ Lyme disease
■ Dermatomyositis
■ Hypersensitivity vasculitis

LABORATORY WORK-UP
■ Skin biopsy
■ Ro/SSA antibody
■ Serum chemistries, looking for evidence of organ dysfunction, particularly kidney, liver & bone marrow

MANAGEMENT
■ Antimalarials
■ Prednisone
■ Thalidomide

SPECIFIC THERAPY
- Hydroxychloroquine 200 mg PO BID
- Prednisone 0.5–1 mg/kg PO QAM
- Thalidomide 100–300 mg PO QD

CAVEATS AND PITFALLS
- Check for possible retinal toxicity w/ hydroxychloroquine every 6 months.
- Consider prednisone or thalidomide only if hydroxychloroquine fails.

LYME DISEASE

ALTERNATE DISEASE NAME
- Lyme borreliosis

HISTORY
- Most cases occur from May to September in endemic areas
- History of tick bite, but often it is not noticed by pt

PHYSICAL EXAMINATION
- Early Lyme disease may begin with flu-like illness
- Erythema migrans
  - Begins as an erythematous macule or papule, often w/ central punctum at site of bite
  - Eruption gradually expands w/ central clearing over days to weeks
  - May have multiple lesions
- Borrelial lymphocytoma: bluish-red nodules, usually on earlobe or nipple
- Acrodermatitis chronica atrophicans
  - Begins as an inflammatory phase marked by edema & erythema, usually on distal extremities
  - Lesions appear on posterior heels & dorsal surfaces of hands, feet, elbows & knees
  - Gradual central progression over months to years
- Systemic involvement
  - Bell's palsy
  - Arthritis

- Chronic fatigue syndrome
- Meningoradiculoneuritis (Bannwarth syndrome) or chronic meningoencephalitis
- Carditis

DIFFERENTIAL DIAGNOSIS
- Insect bite reaction
- Erythema annulare centrifugum
- Granuloma annulare
- Urticaria
- Sarcoidosis
- Tinea corporis
- Seborrheic dermatitis
- Lupus erythematosus
- Benign lymphocytic infiltrate
- Rheumatoid arthritis
- Erythema marginatum rheumaticum
- Psoriatic arthritis
- Reiter syndrome
- Gonococcal arthritis

LABORATORY WORK-UP
- Skin biopsy for histology & culture or polymerase chain reaction (PCR) only if diagnosis is in doubt

MANAGEMENT
- Systemic antibiotics

SPECIFIC THERAPY
- Doxycycline 100 mg PO BID for 10–14 days
- Amoxicillin 500 mg PO TID for 10–14 days
- Erythromycin 250 mg PO QID for 10–14 days

CAVEATS AND PITFALLS
- Most tick bites in endemic areas do not produce Lyme disease; thus, treat only clinically confirmed cases.

LYMPHANGIOMA

ALTERNATE DISEASE NAME
- Cutaneous lymphangioma

- Lymphangioma circumscriptum
- Cavernous lymphangioma
- Cystic hygroma

HISTORY
- First noted at birth or in infancy
- Occasional spontaneous episodes of minor bleeding & copious drainage of clear fluid from ruptured vesicles

PHYSICAL EXAMINATION
- Lymphangioma circumscriptum
  - Small clusters of vesicles, varying in color from pink to red to black (secondary to hemorrhage)
  - May have verrucous surface
- Cavernous lymphangioma: rubbery, multilobulated subcutaneous nodules
- Cystic hygroma: large, soft, translucent cystic lesion, usually occurring in neck, axilla & parotid area

DIFFERENTIAL DIAGNOSIS
- Lymphangiectasia
- Branchiogenic cyst
- Thyroglossal duct cyst
- Herpes simplex virus infection
- Herpes zoster
- Wart
- Epidermoid cyst
- Lipoma
- Hemangioma
- Neurofibroma
- Epidermal nevus
- Melanoma

LABORATORY WORK-UP
- Lesional biopsy

MANAGEMENT
- Complete surgical excision
- Laser ablation
- Cryotherapy

- Sclerotherapy
- Electrocautery

SPECIFIC THERAPY
- See "Management"

CAVEATS AND PITFALLS
- Recurrences common after incomplete removal.

LYMPHOGRANULOMA VENEREUM

ALTERNATE DISEASE NAME
- Lymphogranuloma inguinale
- Climatic bubo
- Nicholas Favre disease

HISTORY
- Sexually transmitted disease
- Associated w/ unprotected sex, anal intercourse, sex w/ partners in endemic countries & multiple sex partners

PHYSICAL EXAMINATION
- Primary stage
  - Small, painless papule or herpetiform ulcer, usually on glans penis or vaginal wall
  - Heals within a few days
- Secondary stage
  - Unilateral painful inguinal lymphadenopathy
  - Horizontal group of inguinal nodes most commonly involved
  - Enlargement of nodes above & below inguinal ligament (groove sign)
- Tertiary stage
  - Proctocolitis, perirectal abscess, fistulas & anal strictures, w/ hyperplasia of intestinal & perirectal lymphatics
  - End result may be elephantiasis of female genitalia, characterized by fibrotic labial thickening, or elephantiasis & deformation of penis in men

DIFFERENTIAL DIAGNOSIS
- Chancroid
- Syphilis

- Granuloma inguinale
- Cat-scratch disease
- Infectious mononucleosis
- Tuberculosis
- Tularemia
- Brucellosis
- Bubonic plague
- Lymphoma
- Metastasis
- Crohn disease

LABORATORY WORK-UP
- Culture aspirate from involved lymph node for chlamydia

MANAGEMENT
- Systemic antibiotics

SPECIFIC THERAPY
- Doxycycline 100 mg PO BID for 3 weeks
- Erythromycin 500 mg PO QID for 3 weeks

CAVEATS AND PITFALLS
- Check for other sexually transmitted diseases.
- Antibiotic therapy does not reverse scarring changes.

LYMPHOMATOID GRANULOMATOSIS

ALTERNATE DISEASE NAME
- Angiocentric lymphoproliferative lesion
- Polymorphic reticulosis

HISTORY
- Systemic multiorgan disease w/ signs & symptoms reflective of organs involved
- Associated w/ Sjögren syndrome, chronic viral hepatitis, rheumatoid arthritis, renal transplantation, human immune deficiency virus (HIV)

PHYSICAL EXAMINATION

- Skin
  - ➤ Patchy, occasionally painful, erythematous macules, papules & plaques involving gluteal regions & extremities
  - ➤ Subcutaneous nodules, which may ulcerate
- Pulmonary: cough; dyspnea; hemoptysis; sputum production, which may reflect associated pneumonia
- Nervous system
  - ➤ Lymphocytic infiltration of meninges, cerebral vessels & peripheral nerves
  - ➤ Mass lesions
  - ➤ Neurologic manifestations include mental status changes, ataxia, hemiparesis, seizures, distal sensory neuropathy, mononeuritis multiplex
- Lethal midline granuloma variant: destructive lesions of midface, nasal cavity, nasal sinuses

DIFFERENTIAL DIAGNOSIS

- Bronchocentric granulomatosis
- Churg-Strauss disease
- Sarcoidosis
- Wegener's granulomatosis
- Non-Hodgkin's lymphoma

LABORATORY WORK-UP

- No diagnostic tests
- Chest radiograph, CBC, chemistry profile as part of general work-up

MANAGEMENT

- Systemic corticosteroids w/ or w/out chemotherapy

SPECIFIC THERAPY

- Prednisone 0.5–1 mg/kg PO QAM until there is objective response

CAVEATS AND PITFALLS

- If prednisone is to be used for >21 days per course of therapy, obtain baseline chest radiograph, TB skin test & bone mineral density determination.

LYMPHOMATOID PAPULOSIS

ALTERNATE DISEASE NAME
- Macaulay disease
- Macaulay's disease

HISTORY
- Gradual onset of an asymptomatic to mildly pruritic papular eruption
- Lesions appear in crops & resolve after several weeks

PHYSICAL EXAMINATION
- Crops of mildly pruritic red papules evolving into red-brown, often hemorrhagic vesicles or pustules w/ necrotic crust, which heal w/ depressed scars
- Most common distribution is on trunk & extremities

DIFFERENTIAL DIAGNOSIS
- Pityriasis lichenoides et varioliformis acuta
- Pseudolymphoma
- Scabies
- Leukemia cutis
- Drug eruption
- Cutaneous B-cell lymphoma
- Hodgkin disease
- Insect bite reaction
- Langerhans cell histiocytosis
- Miliaria
- Folliculitis

LABORATORY WORK-UP
- Skin biopsy, preferably from 2 separate lesions

MANAGEMENT
- Phototherapy or photochemotherapy

SPECIFIC THERAPY
- Methotrexate 5–10 mg PO Q 1 week

CAVEATS AND PITFALLS
- May occasionally develop lymphoreticular malignancy .

MALIGNANT CARCINOID SYNDROME

ALTERNATE DISEASE NAME
- Carcinoid syndrome

HISTORY
- Primary GI tumor often is asymptomatic but may present as acute appendicitis or chronic pain of right quadrant of abdomen
- Cutaneous findings only after metastasis of primary tumor
- Diarrhea & flushing are common presenting signs

PHYSICAL EXAMINATION
- Flushing of face & neck, which may be brief (eg, 2–5 min) or last for several hours
- Fixed telangiectasia and/or violaceous hue, primarily on face & neck, most marked in malar area

DIFFERENTIAL DIAGNOSIS
- Pheochromocytoma
- Mastocytosis
- Pellagra
- Urticaria
- Anaphylaxis
- Angioedema

LABORATORY WORK-UP
- 24-hour urine collection for 5-HIAA

MANAGEMENT
- Systemic antihistamines for symptomatic relief
- Octreotide
- Various cancer chemotherapy regimens

SPECIFIC THERAPY
- Octreotide 100 mcg subcutaneously 3 or 4 times per day

CAVEATS AND PITFALLS
- Certain foods & drugs can complicate interpretation of 5-HIAA determination.

MASTOCYTOSIS

ALTERNATE DISEASE NAME
- Urticaria pigmentosa
- Mastocytosis syndrome

HISTORY
- Most common in children
- Pts w/ widespread cutaneous disease may have acute systemic symptoms exacerbated by physical activity or ingestion of certain drugs or foods
- Systemic symptoms include flushing, wheezing, headache, dyspnea, rhinorrhea, nausea, vomiting, diarrhea & syncope

PHYSICAL EXAMINATION
- Reddish-brown macule or papule that becomes a wheal when rubbed (Darier's sign)
- Solitary mastocytoma
  - First noted within first month of life
  - Rubbery, yellow to brown plaques, urticating w/ or w/out vesiculation after rubbing (bullous urticaria pigmentosa)
- Telangiectasia macularis eruptiva perstans
  - Brown macules & telangiectasias w/ erythema, often over upper trunk
  - Associated w/ peptic ulcer disease
- Diffuse mastocytosis
  - Bullae in infancy, replaced by doughy skin, w/ generalized pruritus; dermatographism, vesicles after minor skin trauma
  - Mast cell infiltration of liver, spleen, skeleton, GI tract
  - Flushing syndrome, most common in early life

DIFFERENTIAL DIAGNOSIS
- Spitz nevus
- Juvenile xanthogranuloma
- Nevus
- Lentigo
- Amyloidosis
- Sarcoidosis
- Granuloma annulare

- Insect bite reaction
- Jessner lymphocytic infiltrate
- Fixed drug eruption
- Lymphoma
- Berloque dermatitis
- Langerhans cell histiocytosis

LABORATORY WORK-UP
- Stroke lesion, looking for urtication
- Skin biopsy w/ mast cell stains

MANAGEMENT
- Systemic antihistamines
- Topical corticosteroids
- Phototherapy

SPECIFIC THERAPY
- Doxepin 10–25 mg PO HS
- Clobetasol 0.05 w% cream applied BID

CAVEATS AND PITFALLS
- Most lesions in children are self-limited & do not require therapy, unless symptomatic.

MEDIAN NAIL DYSTROPHY

ALTERNATE DISEASE NAME
- Median canal dystrophy

HISTORY
- Insidious onset of nail dystrophy over one or more nails
- May appear after nail matrix trauma

PHYSICAL EXAMINATION
- Longitudinal split appearing in center of nail plate, w/ several fine cracks projecting from the line laterally, giving the appearance of a fir tree
- Thumb most often affected
- Spontaneous remission possible after months to years, sometimes w/ recurrences

DIFFERENTIAL DIAGNOSIS
- Underlying anatomic defects, including mucous cyst, squamous cell carcinoma; melanoma; wart or exostosis
- Onychomycosis
- Psoriasis
- Lichen planus

LABORATORY WORK-UP
- None

MANAGEMENT
- No effective therapy

SPECIFIC THERAPY
- None

CAVEATS AND PITFALLS
- None

MELANOMA

ALTERNATE DISEASE NAME
- Malignant melanoma
- Malignant mole

HISTORY
- Occurs most commonly on trunk in white males & lower legs & back in white females
- In pigmented races most common sites are plantar foot, subungual, palmar & mucosal sites.
- Increased risk in large congenital nevi
- Increased risk in pts w/ many nevi or w/ atypical moles & family history of melanoma

PHYSICAL EXAMINATION
- Superficial spreading subtype
  - Flat or slightly elevated papule or plaque, w/ variegate pigmentation (black, brown, blue or pink discoloration)
  - Usually >6 mm in diameter
  - Irregular asymmetric borders

- Nodular subtype
  - Rapid growth of a dark-brown to black papule or dome-shaped nodule, which may be friable & ulcerate
- Lentigo maligna melanoma
  - Arises from intraepithelial precursor lesion, lentigo maligna
  - Slow-growing, irregular, pigmented patch, located on the sun-damaged skin of head, neck & arms of fair-skinned older individuals
  - Evolves into dark-brown to black plaque, which may have raised blue-black papules
- Acral lentiginous subtype
  - Appears on palms, soles or beneath nail plate
  - Subungual lesion presents as diffuse nail discoloration or longitudinal pigmented band within the nail plate, w/ pigment spreading to proximal or lateral nail fold (Hutchinson sign)

DIFFERENTIAL DIAGNOSIS

- Melanocytic nevus, including Clark's nevus (atypical mole, dysplastic nevus)
- Lentigo
- Seborrheic keratosis
- Pyogenic granuloma
- Basal cell carcinoma
- Squamous cell carcinoma
- Dermatofibroma
- Cherry hemangioma
- Metastasis
- Keratoacanthoma
- Chronic paronychia
- Subungual hematoma
- Melanonychia striata

LABORATORY WORK-UP

- Lesional biopsy, w/ complete removal w/out margins, if possible
- Evaluation for possible metastatic disease only if there are localizing signs and/or symptoms

MANAGEMENT

- Wide local excision

- Debatable whether sentinel node biopsy is indicated for melanomas <1 mm or >4 mm thick
- Interferon for high-risk cases

SPECIFIC THERAPY
- See "Management"

CAVEATS AND PITFALLS
- Elective lymph nose dissection of little survival value.
- Sentinel node biopsy indicated only to stage disease.
- Value of interferon in high-risk cases is debatable.

MENINGOCOCCEMIA

ALTERNATE DISEASE NAME
- Meningococcal sepsis

HISTORY
- May follow upper respiratory infection
- Prodrome of headache, nausea, vomiting, myalgias & arthralgias
- With fulminant disease, hypotension & cardiac failure may be apparent within hours of initial presentation

PHYSICAL EXAMINATION
- Early-onset petechiae on extremities & trunk; sometimes progressing to involve any part of body
- With progression, pustules, bullae & hemorrhagic plaques appear, w/ central necrosis & stellate purpura & a "gunmetal gray" hue
- Neurologic findings include headache; altered mental status; neck stiffness; irritability; seizures; nerve palsies; gait disturbance

DIFFERENTIAL DIAGNOSIS
- Bacterial sepsis other than that caused by *Neisseria meningitidis*, such as gonococcemia, *Haemophilus influenzae*, *Streptococcus pneumoniae*; Rocky Mountain spotted fever
- Viral illnesses, especially enteroviruses
- Toxic shock syndrome
- Leptospirosis

- Hypersensitivity vasculitis
- Henoch-Schönlein purpura
- Polyarteritis nodosa
- Dermatomyositis
- Lupus erythematosus
- Coagulopathies, including idiopathic purpura fulminans

LABORATORY WORK-UP
- Blood cultures
- Lumbar puncture
- Skin biopsy for routine histology, Gram stain & culture, although the organism is not often successfully cultured from these lesions

MANAGEMENT
- Systemic antibiotics

SPECIFIC THERAPY
- Penicillin G in sensitive strains: 300,000 U/kg per day, up to 24 million U per day in 4–6 divided doses until 5–7 days after temperature has returned to normal
- Ceftriaxone 2 g or IM q12h until 5–7 days after temperature has returned to normal
- Cefotaxime: for adults, 1–2 g or IM q6–12h; for children <50 kg, 50 mg/kg or IM q8h

CAVEATS AND PITFALLS
- Medical emergency that requires immediate antibiotic therapy while cultures are pending & even before diagnosis is certain.

MERKEL CELL CARCINOMA

ALTERNATE DISEASE NAME
- Trabecular carcinoma
- Small cell carcinoma of skin
- Primary cutaneous neuroendocrine carcinoma

HISTORY
- More common in pts w/ fair skin
- Most common in seventh decade & older
- Increased incidence in immunocompromised pts

PHYSICAL EXAMINATION
- Slow-growing, asymptomatic single, painless, firm, shiny, red or violaceous papule, most commonly in head & neck region & extremities
- Regional nodal metastases first site of dissemination

DIFFERENTIAL DIAGNOSIS
- Squamous cell carcinoma
- Basal cell carcinoma
- Melanoma
- Metastasis
- Kaposi's sarcoma
- Hemangioma
- Dermatofibroma
- Lymphoma

LABORATORY WORK-UP
- Lesional biopsy

MANAGEMENT
- Wide local excision
- Mohs micrographic surgery
- Regional lymph node dissection
- Radiation therapy for local palliation

SPECIFIC THERAPY
- See "Management"

CAVEATS AND PITFALLS
- High rate of recurrence w/ incomplete removal of tumor

MILIARIA

ALTERNATE DISEASE NAME
- Prickly heat
- Sudamina
- Heat rash
- Lichen tropicus
- Tropical anhidrosis

HISTORY
- Miliaria crystallina
  - Usually affects neonates & adults who are febrile or who recently moved to a tropical climate
  - Appears within days to weeks of exposure to hot weather & disappears within hours to days
- Miliaria rubra: typically affects neonates & adults who live in hot, humid environments
- Miliaria profunda: appears in those who live in a tropical climate & have had repeated episodes of miliaria rubra

PHYSICAL EXAMINATION
- Miliaria crystallina
  - Asymptomatic, clear, superficial vesicles appearing in crops, often confluent, & w/out surrounding erythema
  - Lesions rupture easily & resolve w/ superficial, branny desquamation
  - In infants, lesions appear on head, neck & upper part of trunk
  - In adults, lesions occur on trunk
- Miliaria rubra
  - Pruritic or painful, small, discrete, nonfollicular, erythematous papules & vesicles
  - In infants, lesions appear on neck & in groin & axillae
  - In adults, lesions occur on covered skin subject to friction, such as neck, scalp, upper part of trunk & flexures
- Miliaria profunda
  - Asymptomatic, firm, flesh-colored papules, usually on trunk, developing within minutes or hours after stimulation of sweating & resolving quickly after removal of stimulus that caused sweating
  - Increased sweating in unaffected skin
  - Lymphadenopathy
  - Hyperpyrexia & symptoms of heat exhaustion, including dizziness, nausea, dyspnea, palpitations

DIFFERENTIAL DIAGNOSIS
- Folliculitis
- Milia
- Viral exanthem

- Cutaneous candidiasis
- Erythema toxicum
- Insect bite reaction
- Scabies
- Foreign body reaction
- Drug eruption
- Cholinergic urticaria

LABORATORY WORK-UP
- None

MANAGEMENT
- Miliaria crystallina: no therapy indicated
- Miliaria rubra
  - Remove occlusive clothing
  - Limit activity
  - Confine to air-conditioned environment for a few days
- Miliaria profunda
  - Remove occlusive clothing
  - Limit activity
  - Confine to air-conditioned environment for a few days

SPECIFIC THERAPY
- None

CAVEATS AND PITFALLS
- None

MILIUM

ALTERNATE DISEASE NAME
- None

HISTORY
- May arise de novo or after blistering trauma
- Blistering diseases associated w/ milia include bullous pemphigoid, inherited & acquired epidermolysis bullosa, bullous lichen planus, porphyria cutanea tarda & burns

PHYSICAL EXAMINATION
- Uniform, pearly white to yellowish, small, domed papules, often in groups
- Primary milia
  - > Usually on face of newborns
  - > Seen around eye in children & adults
- Secondary lesions: appear after blistering or trauma

DIFFERENTIAL DIAGNOSIS
- Acne vulgaris
- Flat wart
- Syringoma
- Trichoepithelioma
- Xanthoma

LABORATORY WORK-UP
- None

MANAGEMENT
- Incision & drainage
- Destruction w/ light hyfrecation

SPECIFIC THERAPY
- See "Management"

CAVEATS AND PITFALLS
- None

MOLLUSCUM CONTAGIOSUM

ALTERNATE DISEASE NAME
- Water wart
- Molluscum; molluscum sebaceum
- Epithelioma contagiosum

HISTORY
- Most common in young children
- May be sexually transmitted disease
- Widespread, persistent lesions occurring in immunocompromised pts, particularly those w/ HIV disease

PHYSICAL EXAMINATION

- Solitary or grouped, asymptomatic, firm, smooth, umbilicated papules on skin & mucosal surfaces
- Papules may coalesce into plaques
- Self-limited, but may persist for months to years

DIFFERENTIAL DIAGNOSIS

- Wart
- Nevocellular nevus
- Milia
- Syringoma
- Varicella
- Fibrous papule of face
- Basal cell carcinoma
- Sebaceous gland hyperplasia
- Xanthoma
- Juvenile xanthogranuloma
- Epidermoid cyst
- Granuloma annulare
- Cryptococcosis
- Histoplasmosis

LABORATORY WORK-UP

- Potassium hydroxide preparation of lesion contents, looking for grape-like clusters

MANAGEMENT

- Cryotherapy
- Light curettage
- Irritants such as topical retinoids or benzoyl peroxide
- Topical cidofovir for disseminated disease in immunocompromised pts

SPECIFIC THERAPY

- Tretinoin 0.1% cream applied QD for weeks
- Benzoyl peroxide 10% gel applied BID
- Cidofovir 0.3% gel applied twice daily for 7–14 days

CAVEATS AND PITFALLS

- Avoid traumatic treatments in small children, since lesions will eventually self-resolve.

MONGOLIAN SPOT

ALTERNATE DISEASE NAME
- Congenital dermal melanocytosis

HISTORY
- Present at birth
- Most common in darkly pigmented races & in Asians

PHYSICAL EXAMINATION
- Asymptomatic, blue-gray, macular hyperpigmentation, most commonly involving the lumbosacral area, but also buttocks, flanks & shoulder
- Most lesions resolve in early childhood, but some remain for many years

DIFFERENTIAL DIAGNOSIS
- Nevus of Ota/Ito
- Blue nevus
- Child abuse

LABORATORY WORK-UP
- None

MANAGEMENT
- No therapy is indicated

SPECIFIC THERAPY
- None

CAVEATS AND PITFALLS
- None

MORPHEA

ALTERNATE DISEASE NAME
- Localized scleroderma
- Circumscribed scleroderma

HISTORY
- Usually not associated w/ any systemic disease
- Gradual onset of mostly asymptomatic lesions

PHYSICAL EXAMINATION

- Starts as poorly defined areas of nonpitting edema, w/ induration developing as disease progresses
- Skin surface becomes smooth & shiny, w/ loss of hair follicles & decreased ability to sweat
- After months to years, skin softens & becomes atrophic
- Guttate variant: small, white, minimally indurated papules
- Linear variant: discrete, indurated, linear, hypopigmented, sclerotic bands
- Frontoparietal linear morphea (en coup de sabre): linear, atrophic plaque, suggestive of a stroke from a sword, sometimes eventuating in hemifacial atrophy
- Progressive hemifacial atrophy (Romberg-Perry syndrome)
  - ➤ Primary lesion occurs in subcutaneous tissue, muscle & bone
  - ➤ The dermis is affected only secondarily & the skin is not sclerotic
- Eosinophilic fasciitis: acute onset of painful, indurated skin, usually of the upper extremity, w/ orange-peel appearance & swelling of the affected extremity, since the process is in the deep muscle fascia
- Diffuse variant: widespread hypopigmented, sclerotic plaques, often involving upper trunk, abdomen, buttocks, thighs

DIFFERENTIAL DIAGNOSIS

- Lichen sclerosus
- Necrobiosis lipoidica
- Granuloma annulare
- Graft-versus-host disease
- Porphyria cutanea tarda
- Hypertrophic scar
- Progressive systemic sclerosis
- Mixed connective disease
- Lipodermatosclerosis
- Medication- or chemical-induced scleroderma
- Radiation fibrosis
- Scleromyxedema
- Werner syndrome
- Phenylketonuria

LABORATORY WORK-UP
- Lesional biopsy only if diagnosis is in doubt

MANAGEMENT
- Localized disease: no effective therapy
- Diffuse or symptomatic disease
  - Physical therapy
  - Phototherapy
  - Plasmapheresis

SPECIFIC THERAPY
- Methotrexate 5–15 mg PO 1/wk

CAVEATS AND PITFALLS
- No overly effective therapies are available.

MUIR-TORRE SYNDROME

ALTERNATE DISEASE NAME
- Torre syndrome

HISTORY
- Associated w/ one or more visceral malignancies, most commonly colorectal cancer or GU malignancies
- Neoplasms may precede or follow the onset of sebaceous tumors, including sebaceous adenoma, sebaceous epithelioma or sebaceous carcinoma

PHYSICAL EXAMINATION
- One or more flesh-colored to yellow papules, often on face
- Other cutaneous neoplasms include keratoacanthoma, squamous cell carcinoma, multiple follicular cysts

DIFFERENTIAL DIAGNOSIS
- Gardner syndrome
- Cowden syndrome
- Multiple trichoepitheliomas
- Basal cell nevus syndrome
- Basal cell carcinoma

- Squamous cell carcinoma
- Eruptive keratoacanthomas
- Tuberous sclerosis

LABORATORY WORK-UP
- Lesional biopsy
- Work-up for internal malignancy, guided by localizing signs or symptoms

MANAGEMENT
- Surgical excision of sebaceous neoplasms

SPECIFIC THERAPY
- See "Management"

CAVEATS AND PITFALLS
- Suspect GI, lung & GU malignancies, even w/ one sebaceous neoplasm.

MULTICENTRIC RETICULOHISTIOCYTOSIS

ALTERNATE DISEASE NAME
- Lipoid dermatoarthritis
- Lipoid rheumatism
- Giant cell reticulohistiocytosis

HISTORY
- Associated w/ arthritis, which may be presenting sign & sometimes only sign of disease

PHYSICAL EXAMINATION
- Asymptomatic or slightly pruritic, skin-colored or reddish-brown papules or nodules, usually on upper portion of body
- May be isolated from one another or may be clustered, sometimes giving a cobblestone appearance
- Remission possible after years of activity

DIFFERENTIAL DIAGNOSIS
- Rheumatoid nodule
- Xanthoma

- Dermatofibroma
- Progressive nodular histiocytoma
- Juvenile xanthogranuloma
- Leprosy
- Granuloma anulare
- Jessner's lymphocytic infiltration
- Lupus erythematosus
- Langerhans cell histiocytosis
- Lipogranulomatosis
- Gouty tophi
- Sarcoidosis
- Osteoarthritis
- Psoriatic arthritis
- Reiter disease

LABORATORY WORK-UP
- Lesional biopsy
- Radiograph of affected joints

MANAGEMENT
- Phototherapy or photochemotherapy
- Intralesional corticosteroids for localized disease
- Antimalarial agents
- Methotrexate

SPECIFIC THERAPY
- Prednisone
- Triamcinolone, intralesional
- Hydroxychloroquine
- Methotrexate

CAVEATS AND PITFALLS
- If prednisone is to be used for >21 days per course of therapy, obtain baseline chest radiograph, TB skin test & bone mineral density determination.
- Check for possible retinal toxicity w/ hydroxychloroquine every 6 months.

MYIASIS

ALTERNATE DISEASE NAME
- None

HISTORY
- Associated w/ bite of botfly, which leads to deposition of larva in skin

PHYSICAL EXAMINATION
- Wound variant: superficial inflammatory reaction on surface
- Furuncular (follicular) variant: larvae penetrate into skin & produce pruritic inflammatory nodule w/ volcano-like central punctum w/ intermittent exudate

DIFFERENTIAL DIAGNOSIS
- Tungiasis
- Furuncle
- Leishmaniasis
- Inflamed epidermoid cyst
- Insect bite reaction
- Foreign body granuloma
- Atypical mycobacterial infection
- Anthrax
- Nocardia infection

LABORATORY WORK-UP
- Remove & examine contents of lesion under low-power microscopy

MANAGEMENT
- Surgical excision
- Inject lidocaine beneath lesion, then move organism into punctum; make a superficial incision followed by gentle pressure, inward & downward
- Apply bacon fat adjacent to punctum
  - Apply petroleum jelly over punctum

SPECIFIC THERAPY
- See "Management"

CAVEATS AND PITFALLS
- Incomplete removal associated w/ high rate of recurrence.

NECROBIOSIS LIPOIDICA

ALTERNATE DISEASE NAME
- Necrobiosis lipoidica diabeticorum

HISTORY
- Many pts have a personal or family history of diabetes mellitus
- Slowly evolving asymptomatic skin lesions

PHYSICAL EXAMINATION
- Well-circumscribed papule or nodule that expands w/ active border, usually over pretibial area but sometimes arising on face, trunk or extremities
- Evolves into waxy, atrophic, round plaque beginning w/ red-brown color but progressing to yellow-brown color
- May develop painful ulcerations after weeks to months

DIFFERENTIAL DIAGNOSIS
- Morphea
- Lichen sclerosus
- Necrobiotic xanthogranuloma
- Nodular vasculitis
- Granuloma annulare
- Weber-Christian disease
- Factitial disease
- Sarcoidosis
- Xanthoma

LABORATORY WORK-UP
- Lesional biopsy
- Work-up for diabetes mellitus, as baseline

MANAGEMENT
- Topical corticosteroids
- Intralesional corticosteroids
- Aspirin & dipyridamole
- Pentoxifylline

SPECIFIC THERAPY
- Fluocinonide 0.05% cream applied BID

- Triamcinolone 3–4 mg/mL intralesional; advise about possible skin atrophy
- Aspirin 325 mg PO QD & dipyridamole 75 mg PO QID
- Pentoxifylline 400 mg PO TID

CAVEATS AND PITFALLS
- Generally poor response to therapy, even w/ good control of diabetes mellitus.

NECROTIZING FASCIITIS

ALTERNATE DISEASE NAME
- Hospital gangrene
- Acute infective gangrene
- Necrotizing erysipelas
- Suppurative fasciitis

HISTORY
- Explosive onset of multisystem disorder w/ rapidly deteriorating organ functions
- Typically occurs after trauma, surgical wound or hematogenous seeding from another infection site

PHYSICAL EXAMINATION
- Most commonly involves extremities or trunk, but may involve perineum (Fornier's gangrene)
- Early, severe, local pain, out of proportion to visible findings
- Poorly marginated red plaque w/ subcutaneous edema, which progresses to dusky plaque w/ vesiculation & occasional crepitus
- Marked constitutional changes including fever, prostration, decreased sensorium & hypotension

DIFFERENTIAL DIAGNOSIS
- Cellulitis
- Sweet syndrome
- Pyoderma gangrenosum
- Polyarteritis nodosa or other vasculitides
- Insect envenomation
- Vascular insufficiency

LABORATORY WORK-UP
- Wound Gram stain & culture
- Blood cultures

MANAGEMENT
- Surgical debridement
- Systemic antibiotics

SPECIFIC THERAPY
- Penicillin G 8–10 million units IV, given q4–6h
- Clindamycin 600–900 mg IV q6–12h

CAVEATS AND PITFALLS
- Surgical emergency; needs immediate debridement.

NEVUS ANEMICUS

ALTERNATE DISEASE NAME
- None

HISTORY
- Present at birth, but may be difficult to discern because of similarity of color to background
- Increased frequency in pts w/ neurofibromatosis

PHYSICAL EXAMINATION
- Permanent, irregularly shaped, pale patch, w/ stellate margins
- Usually located on upper trunk

DIFFERENTIAL DIAGNOSIS
- Nevus depigmentosus
- Hypomelanosis of Ito
- Segmental vitiligo
- Tinea versicolor
- Postinflammatory hypopigmentation
- Leprosy
- Tuberous sclerosis

LABORATORY WORK-UP
- Ice cube test: place ice cube on lesion; positive test is when lesion does not turn red after ice cube is removed

MANAGEMENT
- None

SPECIFIC THERAPY
- None

CAVEATS AND PITFALLS
- None

NEVUS FLAMMEUS

ALTERNATE DISEASE NAME
- Nevus flammeus neonatorum
- Port-wine stain
- Port-wine mark
- Strawberry patch

HISTORY
- Present at birth, but may not be apparent early in life because of similar skin color in some newborns

PHYSICAL EXAMINATION
- Pink to violaceous patch, w/ variable blanching after external pressure
- Typically located over head & neck area
- Surface may become thickened w/ a cobblestone-like contour & vascular papules or nodules or pyogenic granuloma-like lesions, usually in adulthood
- Skin & underlying soft tissue or bony hypertrophy may occur
- Sturge-Weber (encephalofacial or encephalotrigeminal angiomatosis) variant
  - Vascular malformations involving the upper facial area supplied by ophthalmic branch (CN V1) of the trigeminal nerve, the ipsilateral leptomeninges & the ipsilateral cerebral cortex
  - More extensive than in isolated nevus flammeus
  - Complications include glaucoma, seizures, hemiplegia, mental retardation, cerebral calcifications, subdural hemorrhage & underlying soft tissue hypertrophy

DIFFERENTIAL DIAGNOSIS
- Salmon patch

- Capillary hemangioma
- Beckwith-Wiedemann syndrome
- Coats disease
- Cobb syndrome
- Parkes-Weber syndrome
- Phakomatosis pigmentovascularis
- von Hippel-Lindau disease
- Wyburn-Mason syndrome

LABORATORY WORK-UP
- None

MANAGEMENT
- Flashlamp-pumped pulsed dye laser

SPECIFIC THERAPY
- See "Management"

CAVEATS AND PITFALLS
- Work-up for CNS involvement only if there are localizing signs & symptoms.

NEVUS OF OTA AND ITO

ALTERNATE DISEASE NAME
- Oculodermal melanosis
- Nevus fuscoceruleus zygomaticus
- Hori's nevus
- Hori nevus
- Nevus fuscoceruleus acromiodeltoideus
- Nevus fuscoceruleus ophthalmomaxillaris

HISTORY
- Present at birth, but may be inapparent during newborn period
- May slowly progress by darkening & enlarging, but is stable after adulthood reached

PHYSICAL EXAMINATION
- Nevus of Ota
  - Usually unilateral, poorly demarcated, gray-blue patch over cheek, forehead, eyelid, temple & gingiva

> ➤ Sclera blue & shiny
> ➤ Distribution may follow the 2 first branches of the trigeminal nerve
■ Nevus of Ito: same appearance & course as nevus of Ota, but located over shoulder & upper arm areas

DIFFERENTIAL DIAGNOSIS
■ Blue nevus
■ Melasma
■ Ochronosis
■ Melanoma
■ Lentigo
■ Traumatic tattoo

LABORATORY WORK-UP
■ None

MANAGEMENT
■ Q-switched ruby, Q-switched alexandrite or Q-switched Nd:YAG laser ablation

SPECIFIC THERAPY
■ See "Management"

CAVEATS AND PITFALLS
■ Rare malignant degeneration, but base treatment decisions only on cosmetic considerations.

NEVUS SPILUS

ALTERNATE DISEASE NAME
■ Speckled lentiginous nevus
■ Speckled nevus spilus
■ Mosaic speckled lentiginous nevus
■ Nevus on nevus

HISTORY
■ Present at birth
■ Enlarges in proportion to normal growth

PHYSICAL EXAMINATION
- Variable number of black, brown or red-brown macules & flat papules seen within oval or linear (zosteriform) patch of tan to brown hyperpigmentation
- May follow lines of Blaschko

DIFFERENTIAL DIAGNOSIS
- Congenital melanocytic nevus
- Spitz nevus
- NAME syndrome
- LEOPARD syndrome
- Carney's syndrome

LABORATORY WORK-UP
- None

MANAGEMENT
- Surgical removal
- Laser ablation w/ Q-switched ruby or Q-switched Nd:YAG laser

SPECIFIC THERAPY
- See "Management"

CAVEATS AND PITFALLS
- Treatment for cosmetic reasons only.

NEVUS, MELANOCYTIC

ALTERNATE DISEASE NAME
- Nevocellular nevus
- Mole

HISTORY
- Congenital variant
  - Present from birth w/ slow enlargement & thickening over first few years of life, in many cases
  - Large lesions are at greater risk for melanoma.
- Clark's nevus variant: family history of melanoma & presence of multiple lesions are melanoma risk factors

PHYSICAL EXAMINATION
- Congenital variant
  - ➣ Size may range from <1 cm to lesions large enough to cover most of the integument
  - ➣ Color may range from tan to deep blue-black.
  - ➣ May start as patch & become palpable as child ages
  - ➣ Associated satellite pigmented papules, especially in pts w/ giant congenital nevus (>20 cm in diameter)
- Acquired variant: sharply marginated, uniform tan to brown, smooth to verrucous papule or macule, usually <1 cm in diameter
- Spitz (spindle cell) nevus variant: usual childhood onset of uniform, smooth, reddish-brown papule, often w/ fine overlying scale
- Blue nevus variant: uniform, firm blue papule
- Clark's nevus (atypical mole, dysplastic nevus) variant: reddish-brown flat papule, w/ central elevation & feathered red border ("fried egg appearance"), often >0.5 cm in diameter

DIFFERENTIAL DIAGNOSIS
- Melanoma
- Seborrheic keratosis
- Nevus of Ota/Ito
- Lentigo
- Freckle
- Benign tumor of sweat gland or hair follicle
- Mastocytoma
- Juvenile xanthogranuloma
- Basal cell carcinoma
- Actinic keratosis

LABORATORY WORK-UP
- Lesional biopsy only if diagnosis is in doubt or if melanoma is a possibility

MANAGEMENT
- Congenital nevus: surgical excision, particularly larger lesions
- Acquired nevus, blue nevus or Spitz nevus: surgical excision

SPECIFIC THERAPY
- See "Management."

CAVEATS AND PITFALLS
- Surgical removal of acquired nevi for cosmetic reasons or for diagnosis
- Controversial whether Clark's nevus should be excised as possible preventive measure against melanoma

NOCARDIOSIS

ALTERNATE DISEASE NAME
- *Nocardia* infection

HISTORY
- Often preceded by skin trauma, such as puncture wound or other minor injury while walking barefoot or working with one's hands

PHYSICAL EXAMINATION
- Superficial skin infection
  - Fever w/out lymphadenopathy
  - Purulent crusting papule that subsequently ulcerates
- Lymphocutaneous infection
  - Begins as ulcerative papule or nodule at inoculation site, often on upper extremities
  - Secondary subcutaneous nodules develop along lymphatic vessels
  - Regional lymphadenopathy
- Disseminated nocardiosis
  - Occurs predominately in immunocompromised pts
  - Pulmonary findings are usually most prominent
  - Local disease associated w/ metastatic abscesses, typically in lower extremities
  - Brain abscess, w/ altered mental status, personality changes, localized neurologic findings; meningitis, altered consciousness & meningismus

DIFFERENTIAL DIAGNOSIS
- Ecthyma
- Cellulitis
- Sporotrichosis
- Atypical mycobacterial infection

- North American blastomycosis
- Coccidioidomycosis
- Leishmaniasis
- Anthrax
- Orf
- Milker's nodule
- Cutaneous tuberculosis
- Herpes simplex virus infection
- Actinomycosis

LABORATORY WORK-UP
- Lesional culture
- Chest radiograph if primary pulmonary nocardiosis is suspected

MANAGEMENT
- Systemic antibiotics

SPECIFIC THERAPY
- Trimethoprim/sulfamethoxazole DS strength BID for at least 3 weeks
- Minocycline 100–200 mg PO BID for 2–4 weeks

CAVEATS AND PITFALLS
- None

NORTH AMERICAN BLASTOMYCOSIS

ALTERNATE DISEASE NAME
- Blastomycosis

HISTORY
- May present as a flu-like illness or as an acute pneumonia
- Chronic disease may simulate tuberculosis or lung cancer, w/ symptoms of low-grade fever, productive cough, night sweats, weight loss
- Usually starts w/ pulmonary infection followed by cutaneous, osseous, GU or CNS involvement

PHYSICAL EXAMINATION

- Skin findings
  - ➤ Lesions usually occur on exposed areas & present as minimally tender papules or pustules.
  - ➤ Lesions evolve into purulent, verrucous or ulcerative nodules or plaques, characterized by sharp & heaped-up borders w/ centrally located granulation tissue & exudate.
- Pulmonary findings
  - ➤ Fever, night sweats, wheezing & dyspnea
  - ➤ Signs & symptoms of chronic pneumonia, lasting for 2–6 months, include weight loss, night sweats, fever, cough, chest pain.
- Other systemic signs include osteolytic bone lesions, prostatitis, epididymitis.

DIFFERENTIAL DIAGNOSIS

- Basal cell carcinoma
- Squamous cell carcinoma
- Pyoderma gangrenosum
- Keratoacanthoma
- Wart
- Leishmaniasis
- Cutaneous anthrax
- Disseminated coccidioidomycosis
- Nocardiosis
- Atypical mycobacterial infection
- Cutaneous tuberculosis
- Sarcoidosis

LABORATORY WORK-UP

- Sputum microscopy & culture
- Microscopic exam of a potassium hydroxide wet mount of pus aspirated or expressed from skin microabscesses, fistula or subcutaneous abscesses
- Lesional biopsy for histology & culture

MANAGEMENT

- Systemic antimycotic therapy for symptomatic disease

SPECIFIC THERAPY

- Amphotericin B 0.7–1 mg/kg IV per day; total dose 1.5–2.5 g
- Itraconazole 200–400 mg PO QD for at least 6 months
- Ketoconazole 400–800 mg PO QD for at least 6 months

CAVEATS AND PITFALLS

- For symptomatic disease, consider oral antimycotic therapy before amphotericin B unless pt is extremely ill.

NOTALGIA PARESTHETICA

ALTERNATE DISEASE NAME

- Paresthetic notalgia

HISTORY

- Paroxysmal intense localized pruritus, usually arising in adulthood & persisting for decades
- Rare early clinical marker of multiple endocrine neoplasia type IIA

PHYSICAL EXAMINATION

- Pruritus, pain and/or paresthesia occurring principally between the scapulas, sometimes attacking either side of the midline or posterolateral aspect of the shoulder
- Hyperpigmentation secondary to chronic rubbing & scratching

DIFFERENTIAL DIAGNOSIS

- Lichen amyloidosis
- Atopic neurodermatitis
- Post-herpetic neuralgia
- Xerosis
- Contact dermatitis
- Intercostal neuralgia
- Thoracic outlet syndrome

LABORATORY WORK-UP

- None

MANAGEMENT

- Capsaicin
- Oxcarbazepine
- Local nerve block

SPECIFIC THERAPY
- Capsaicin 0.075% cream applied 4 or 5 times per day
- Oxcarbazepine 300 mg PO twice daily; titration of dose to effect

CAVEATS AND PITFALLS
- Advise about burning sensation w/ each application of capsaicin.
  - ➤ Consider spinal nerve outlet syndrome.

NUMMULAR ECZEMA

ALTERNATE DISEASE NAME
- Nummular dermatitis
- Discoid eczema

HISTORY
- Seen more frequently in atopic pts
- Exposure to environmental irritants may worsen symptoms
- Skin dryness, temperature changes & stress can worsen symptoms

PHYSICAL EXAMINATION
- Starts as papules or vesicles that coalesce to form confluent plaques on erythematous base
- Lower extremities & dorsum of hand most frequently affected areas
- Early lesions may be exudative & crusted
- Older lesions are dry, scaly & excoriated from scratching

DIFFERENTIAL DIAGNOSIS
- Atopic dermatitis
- Lichen simplex chronicus
- Tinea corporis
- Contact dermatitis
- Psoriasis
- Stasis dermatitis
- Pityriasis lichenoides

LABORATORY WORK-UP
- Lesional biopsy if diagnosis is in doubt

MANAGEMENT
- Topical corticosteroids
- Systemic corticosteroids only in short courses for extreme flares

SPECIFIC THERAPY
- Fluocinonide 0.05% cream applied BID
- Prednisone 1 mg/kg PO QAM for up to 14 days
- Triamcinolone 40–80 mg IM

CAVEATS AND PITFALLS
- Xerosis & atopic dermatitis are most common associated conditions; aggressive therapy of these problems will improve the nummular dermatitis.

OCHRONOSIS

ALTERNATE DISEASE NAME
- Alcaptonuria
- Alkaptonuria
- Homogentisic acid oxidase deficiency

HISTORY
- Dark urine in diapers is usual first sign of disease
- Ochronosis-like pigmentation may occur as a reaction to application of hydroquinone or phenol

PHYSICAL EXAMINATION
- Discoloration on nasal tip, costochondral junctions, extensor tendons of hands, cheeks, fingernails & buccal mucosa
- Gray-black scleral pigmentation in configuration of small, dark rings
- Ear cartilage discoloration w/ a grayish-blue hue, followed by structural changes w/ stiffness, contour irregularities & calcification
- Ochronotic arthropathy

DIFFERENTIAL DIAGNOSIS
- Argyria
- Medication-related hyperpigmentation
- Postinflammatory hyperpigmentation

LABORATORY WORK-UP
- Darkening of urine w/ the addition of sodium hydroxide
- Urine homogentisic acid levels

MANAGEMENT
- No effective therapy

SPECIFIC THERAPY
- None

CAVEATS AND PITFALLS
- Products with a high concentration of hydroquinone may cause ochronosis-like pigmentation, particularly in black pts.

ONYCHOMYCOSIS

ALTERNATE DISEASE NAME
- Fungal nail infection

HISTORY
- Related to nail trauma in some cases
- Most often is asymptomatic & slowly evolving process
- Occasional paresthesia, pain, discomfort & loss of dexterity

PHYSICAL EXAMINATION
- Distal lateral subungual type: thickened & opacified nail plate, nail bed hyperkeratosis & onycholysis
- Endonyx variant: milky-white discoloration of nail plate w/out subungual hyperkeratosis or onycholysis
- Superficial white onychomycosis
  - Small, white speckled or powdery macules on surface of toe-nail plate
  - Nail is roughened & crumbles readily
  - Proximal subungual variant: leukonychia in proximal nail fold
- Candidal infection: paronychia; onycholysis; gross hyperkeratosis of nail bed & inflammation of nail fold in chronic mucocutaneous disease

DIFFERENTIAL DIAGNOSIS
- Psoriasis

- Traumatic nail dystrophy
- Twenty nail dystrophy
- Lichen planus
- Subungual melanoma
- Contact dermatitis
- Pachonychia congenita
- Darier disease
- Nail patella syndrome
- Bacterial paronychia
- Yellow nail syndrome
- Pityriasis rubra pilaris
- Drug-related nail dystrophy

LABORATORY WORK-UP
- Potassium hydroxide preparation of subungual debris, looking for hyphal elements
- Fungal culture of subungual debris

MANAGEMENT
- Systemic & topical antifungal agents
- Surgical nail avulsion & matrix destruction for persistent, symptomatic lesions unresponsive to medical therapy

SPECIFIC THERAPY
- Terbinafine 250 mg PO QD for 3 months
- Itraconazole 200 mg PO BID 1 week per month for 3 months
- Griseofulvin 500 mg PO BID for 6–12 months
- Fluconazole 150 mg PO once weekly for 3–6 months
- Ciclopirox nail lacquer applied BID for at least 48 weeks (12% cure rate)

CAVEATS AND PITFALLS
- Topical forms of therapy are almost never curative.
- High recurrence rate for all forms of therapy.

ORF

ALTERNATE DISEASE NAME
- Sheep-pox
- Contagious ecthyma

- Ecthyma contagiosum
- Ecthyma infectiosum
- Contagious pustular dermatitis

HISTORY
- Occurs about 1 week after contact w/ infected animal
- May be associated w/ low-grade constitutional symptoms

PHYSICAL EXAMINATION
- Small, firm, red to blue papule growing to form hemorrhagic, flat-topped pustule or bulla, w/ crust or central umbilication, on fingers, hands or forearms
- Spontaneous resolution after 30–40 days

DIFFERENTIAL DIAGNOSIS
- Bacterial ecthyma
- Milker's nodule
- Tularemia
- Sporotrichosis
- Nocardiosis
- Anthrax
- Acute febrile neutrophilic dermatosis
- Leishmaniasis
- Cutaneous tuberculosis
- Squamous cell carcinoma
- Keratoacanthoma

LABORATORY WORK-UP
- None

MANAGEMENT
- Surgical excision or destruction by electrodesiccation & curettage for persistent lesion

SPECIFIC THERAPY
- See "Management"

CAVEATS AND PITFALLS
- None

OSLER-WEBER-RENDU DISEASE

ALTERNATE DISEASE NAME
- Hereditary hemorrhagic telangiectasia
- Rendu-Osler syndrome
- Osler's disease
- Osler disease
- Heredofamilial angiomatosis
- Familial hemorrhagic angiomatosis

HISTORY
- Recurrent epistaxis is usual presenting sign
- Risk of GI tract bleeding increases after age 50 years

PHYSICAL EXAMINATION
- Telangiectases found on oral mucosa, nasal mucosa, skin & conjunctiva
- Minute bright red to violaceous, partially blanching macules or barely palpable papules
- Face, lips & mouth, nares, tongue, ears, hands, chest & feet most commonly affected sites
- Cyanosis & clubbing may occur in pts w/ pulmonary AV malformations
- Cerebrovascular accident, brain abscess or intracerebral hematoma w/ CNS involvement
- Pulmonary complications include AV malformations, tachypnea, cyanosis & clubbing
- Retinal telangiectasias & hemorrhages
- GI bleeding

DIFFERENTIAL DIAGNOSIS
- Benign essential telangiectasia
- Rosacea
- Actinically damaged skin
- Ataxia-telangiectasia
- CREST syndrome
- Louis-Bar syndrome
- Dermatomyositis
- Rothmund-Thomson syndrome

- Scleroderma
- Cockayne syndrome
- Angiokeratoma corporis diffusum

LABORATORY WORK-UP
- CBC, platelet count
- Serum iron level
- Stool, urine exam for occult blood

MANAGEMENT
- Laser ablation of symptomatic lesions w/ Nd:YAG laser
- Recurrent, uncontrollable epistaxis: septal dermoplasty
- Bleeding prophylaxis

SPECIFIC THERAPY
- Bleeding prophylaxis: estradiol 0.62502 mg PO per day or via transdermal patch

CAVEATS AND PITFALLS
- None

OTITIS EXTERNA

ALTERNATE DISEASE NAME
- External otitis
- Swimmer's ear

HISTORY
- Related to prolonged water immersion
- Presents w/ otalgia, tinnitus, hearing loss, pruritus & feeling of ear fullness

PHYSICAL EXAMINATION
- Pain on palpation of tragus or when applying traction to pinna
- Edema & redness of ear canal
- Thick white, gray or serous discharge
- Conductive hearing loss
- Necrotizing (malignant) otitis externa variant
  - Pain out of proportion to clinical findings
  - Granulation tissue in ear canal

DIFFERENTIAL DIAGNOSIS
- Otitis media
- Foreign body in ear canal
- Squamous cell carcinoma of ear canal
- Ear canal trauma
- Erysipelas

LABORATORY WORK-UP
- Ear canal bacterial & fungal culture

MANAGEMENT
- Topical antibiotic/corticosteroid solution
- Acetic acid soaks
- Systemic corticosteroids for severe flare
- Surgical debridement for necrotizing variant

SPECIFIC THERAPY
- Neomycin, polymyxin B, hydrocortisone otic solution applied 4 times daily for 10–14 days
- Hydrocortisone & acetic acid otic solution applied on cotton wick 4 times daily for 10–14 days
- Acetic acid 5% in aluminium acetate solution applied on cotton wick 3 or 4 times daily until symptoms abate
- Prednisone 1 mg/kg PO QD for 7–14 days

CAVEATS AND PITFALLS
- Swimming or other immersion activities may prolong course of illness.

PACHYONYCHIA CONGENITA

ALTERNATE DISEASE NAME
- Jadassohn-Lewandowsky syndrome
- Polykeratosis congenita

HISTORY
- Usually noted shortly after birth

PHYSICAL EXAMINATION
- Jadassohn-Lewandowsky type (PC-1)
  - ➤ Thickened, brown to gray nail plates w/ rough surface; usually affecting all fingers

- ➤ Toenails occasionally affected
- ➤ Fingernail involvement may spread into periungual tissue, causing paronychial inflammation
- ➤ Circumscribed or diffuse hyperkeratoses of palms & soles
- ➤ Follicular hyperkeratosis on face & on extensor aspect of proximal extremities
- ➤ Leukokeratosis of oral mucosa
- ■ Jackson-Lawler type (PC-2)
  - ➤ Thickened nail plates & other features of PC-1 type
  - ➤ Natal teeth
  - ➤ Unruly hair

DIFFERENTIAL DIAGNOSIS
- ■ Psoriasis
- ■ Pityriasis rubra pilaris
- ■ Onychomycosis
- ■ Darier disease
- ■ Epidermolysis bullosa
- ■ Mucocutaneous candidiasis

LABORATORY WORK-UP
- ■ Biopsy of oral lesion to rule out carcinoma

MANAGEMENT
- ■ Systemic retinoids

SPECIFIC THERAPY
- ■ Acitretin 25–50 mg PO QD indefinitely

CAVEATS AND PITFALLS
- ■ Systemic retinoids are contraindicated in women of childbearing potential.

PAGET'S DISEASE

ALTERNATE DISEASE NAME
- ■ Paget's disease of nipple & areola
- ■ Paget's disease of skin, apocrine type
- ■ Eczematoid epitheliomatous dermatosis
- ■ Malignant papillary dermatosis
- ■ Intraepidermal adenocarcinoma

HISTORY
- May be first considered after long history of an eczematous skin lesion in the nipple & adjacent areas or in the groin, genitalia, perineum or perianal area

PHYSICAL EXAMINATION
- Mammary variant
  - Sharply demarcated, scaly, red, crusted & thickened plaques on nipple, spreading to surrounding areolar areas
  - May cause retraction of nipple or palpable nodules indicating an underlying breast cancer
  - May have serosanguinous nipple discharge
- Extramammary variant
  - Eczematous plaque leading to a unilateral, sharply marginated lesion w/ peripheral erythema
  - Erosion or scaling may appear in older lesions

DIFFERENTIAL DIAGNOSIS
- Mammary variant
  - Irritant contact dermatitis
  - Atopic dermatitis
  - Fixed drug eruption
  - Nipple duct adenoma
  - Erosive adenomatosis of nipple
  - Melanoma
  - Bowen's disease
- Extramammary variant
  - Lichen simplex chronicus
  - Bowen's disease
  - Basal cell carcinoma
  - Melanoma
  - Candidiasis
  - Intertrigo
  - Contact dermatitis
  - Seborrheic dermatitis
  - Psoriasis

LABORATORY WORK-UP
- Skin biopsy

MANAGEMENT
- Mammary variant: mastectomy & lymph node clearance
- Extramammary variant
  - Surgical excision w/ Mohs micrographic surgery or wide local excision
  - Imiquimod

SPECIFIC THERAPY
- Imiquimod applied 2–3 times weekly for 16 weeks

CAVEATS AND PITFALLS
- May be associated w/ underlying bladder or colon cancer; workup is indicated to rule out these malignancies.

PAPULAR MUCINOSIS

ALTERNATE DISEASE NAME
- Lichen myxedematosus
- Myxedematosus
- Scleromyxedema

HISTORY
- Slow onset of a mildly pruritic eruption
- Pts remain in otherwise good health

PHYSICAL EXAMINATION
- Papular mucinosis (lichen myxedematosus) variant
  - Dome-shaped & flesh-colored or erythematous papules, often in a pattern of parallel ridges
  - Lesions may coalesce into grouped lichenoid papules on dorsal hands, face or extensor surfaces of arms & legs
  - With extensive involvement, leonine facies may develop
- Scleromyxedema variant
  - Widespread, erythematous, indurated skin resembling scleroderma, w/ diffuse tightness & decreased range of motion
  - Systemic manifestations include restrictive & obstructive pulmonary dysfunction, cardiovascular abnormalities & polyarthritis
  - GI symptoms (most commonly dysphagia) related to deficient esophageal peristalsis

➤ Proximal muscle weakness & polyarthritis
➤ Symptoms similar to those of organic brain syndrome
➤ Ectropion & corneal opacities
➤ Cardiovascular abnormalities

DIFFERENTIAL DIAGNOSIS

- Scleroderma
- Scleredema
- Leprosy
- Sarcoidosis
- Persistent acral papular mucinosis
- Malignant atrophic papulosis
- Lymphoma
- Follicular mucinosis
- Darier disease
- Grover's disease
- Colloid milium
- Granuloma annulare
- Scleredema
- Leprosy
- Sarcoidosis
- Lipoid proteinosis
- Progressive nodular histiocytosis

LABORATORY WORK-UP

- Skin biopsy w/ mucin stains
- Serum protein immunoelectrophoresis looking for a serum paraprotein (usually 7S-IgG) w/ lambda light chains

MANAGEMENT

- Systemic retinoids
- Systemic corticosteroids
- Orthovoltage radiation
- Electron beam radiation
- Photochemotherapy
- Plasmapheresis
- Extracorporeal photophoresis
- Dermabrasion
- Laser ablation

SPECIFIC THERAPY
- Acitretin 1 mg/kg PO QD indefinitely
- Prednisone: start with 1 mg/kg/day and titrate as per response to therapy

CAVEATS AND PITFALLS
- If prednisone is to be used for >21 days per course of therapy, obtain baseline chest radiograph, TB skin test & bone mineral density determination.
- Systemic retinoids are contraindicated in women of child-bearing potential.

PARANEOPLASTIC PEMPHIGUS

ALTERNATE DISEASE NAME
- None

HISTORY
- Pre-existing malignancy, most commonly non-Hodgkin's lymphoma, but may include chronic lymphocytic leukemia, Castleman tumor, giant cell lymphoma, Waldenström macroglobulinemia, thymoma, poorly differentiated sarcoma, bronchogenic squamous cell carcinoma or follicular dendritic cell sarcoma
- Associated w/ poor prognosis in many cases

PHYSICAL EXAMINATION
- Oral erosions or ulcerations, occurring anywhere in mouth, usually as first sign of disease
- Erosions in nose, pharynx, tonsils, GI tract, respiratory tract & genital mucosal surfaces
- Variable skin lesions, including diffuse erythema, vesiculobullous lesions, papules, scaly plaques, exfoliative erythroderma, erosions, ulcerations
- Ocular involvement includes conjunctivitis & symblepharon w/ corneal scarring

DIFFERENTIAL DIAGNOSIS
- Erythema multiforme
- Stevens-Johnson syndrome
- Pemphigus vulgaris

- Toxic epidermal necrolysis
- Bullous pemphigoid
- Cicatricial pemphigoid
- Epidermolysis bullosa acquisita
- Lichen planus

LABORATORY WORK-UP
- Skin biopsy for routine histology & direct immunofluorescence

MANAGEMENT
- Systemic corticosteroids
- Corticosteroid-sparing drugs
- Plasmapheresis

SPECIFIC THERAPY
- Prednisone 0.502 mg/kg PO QAM
- Steroid-sparing agents
  - Azathioprine 2–3 mg/kg PO QD
  - Cyclosporine 3–5 mg/kg PO QD
  - Mycophenolate mofetil 2–3 g PO QD
  - Cyclophosphamide 100–200 mg PO QD

CAVEATS AND PITFALLS
- If prednisone is to be used for >21 days per course of therapy, obtain baseline chest radiograph, TB skin test & bone mineral density determination.
- Check thiopurine methyltransferase levels before starting azathioprine therapy.
- Check for possible renal toxicity & hypertension w/ cyclosporine therapy.

PARONYCHIA

ALTERNATE DISEASE NAME
- Finger infection
- Fingernail infection
- Runaround abscess
- Runaround infection

HISTORY
- History of minor nail trauma or manipulation
- Pain, tenderness & swelling in one of the lateral folds of the nail
- With chronic variant, inflammation, pain & swelling occur episodically, often after exposure to moist environment

PHYSICAL EXAMINATION
- Acute variant
  - Erythematous, edematous distal finger, sometimes w/ purulent exudate
  - Most prominent in proximal & lateral nail fold area, w/ extension into eponychium
  - Purulence of nail bed may cause raising of nail plate off bed
- Chronic variant
  - Edematous, erythematous, tender nail folds w/out purulent discharge
  - Thickened & discolored nail plates, w/ transverse ridges

DIFFERENTIAL DIAGNOSIS
- Mucocutaneous candidiasis
- Herpetic whitlow
- Onychomycosis
- Contact dermatitis
- Periungual wart
- Squamous cell carcinoma
- Melanoma

LABORATORY WORK-UP
- Gram stain, KOH preparation of exudate
- Bacterial fungal culture of exudate

MANAGEMENT
- Acute variant
  - Warm water soaks
  - Systemic antibiotics
  - Surgical incision & drainage if abscess forms
- Chronic variant
  - Avoidance of inciting factors such as exposure to moist environments, skin irritants or nail manipulation
  - If *Candida* is causative, topical or systemic antifungal agents
  - Eponychial marsupialization in recalcitrant cases

SPECIFIC THERAPY
- Amoxicillin 250–500 mg PO TID for 10 days
- Clotrimazole 1% cream applied BID for 21 days
- Fluconazole 150 mg PO for 1 dose

CAVEATS AND PITFALLS
- Use systemic antibiotics only for culture-proven bacterial infection.

PEDICULOSIS

ALTERNATE DISEASE NAME
- Lice
- Phthiriasis

HISTORY
- Head lice: intermittent pruritus w/ evidence of excoriation, especially at nape of neck
- Body lice: organisms infest seams of clothing, where nits may be found

PHYSICAL EXAMINATION
- Pediculosis capitis (head lice)
  - Organisms most commonly found in retroauricular scalp
  - Nits attach to hair shafts just above level of scalp
- Pediculosis corporis (body lice): hemosiderin-stained purpuric macules where lice have fed (maculae ceruleae)
- Pediculosis pubis (pubic lice)
  - Lice & nits visible throughout pubic hair, extending onto adjacent hair-bearing areas
  - Same organism infesting eyelashes

DIFFERENTIAL DIAGNOSIS
- Hair casts
- Seborrheic dermatitis
- Acne keloidalis
- Scabies
- Impetigo
- Benign pigmented purpura
- Folliculitis decalvans

LABORATORY WORK-UP
- Microscopic exam of hair, looking for nits

MANAGEMENT
- Topical pediculicidal agent
- Ivermectin

SPECIFIC THERAPY
- Permethrin 1% cream rinse
- Complete nit removal w/ nit comb or chemical remover such as Step 2
- Ivermectin 200 mcg/kg PO for 1 dose

CAVEATS AND PITFALLS
- Incomplete therapy associated w/ high rate of recurrence.
- Other common cause of second infection is re-infection from family member, etc.

PEMPHIGUS FOLIACEUS

ALTERNATE DISEASE NAME
- Superficial pemphigus

HISTORY
- Insidious onset of lesions, occasionally w/ pruritus
- General health unaffected

PHYSICAL EXAMINATION
- Transient, superficial vesicles & bullae, evolving into crusted papules or erosions on an erythematous base, occurring in seborrheic areas, w/ little or no involvement of mucous membranes
- Pemphigus erythematosus (Senear-Usher) variant
  - ➤ Features of lupus erythematosus & pemphigus foliaceus
  - ➤ Red scaly plaques on bridge of nose & malar area
  - ➤ Occasional exfoliative erythroderma as extreme manifestation
- Pemphigus herpetiformis variant
  - ➤ Starts as pruritic grouped papules & vesicles, suggestive of dermatitis herpetiformis
  - ➤ May have occasional oral erosions

- Drug-induced variant: may occur w/ penicillamine or captopril, usually after at least 2 months of use

DIFFERENTIAL DIAGNOSIS

- Pemphigus vulgaris
- Paraneoplastic pemphigus
- Bullous pemphigoid
- Erythema multiforme
- Transient acantholytic dermatosis
- Hailey-Hailey disease
- Subcorneal pustular dermatosis
- Dermatitis herpetiformis
- Linear IgA dermatosis
- Lupus erythematosus
- Impetigo
- Darier disease

LABORATORY WORK-UP

- Biopsy of fresh lesion for routine histology
- Biopsy of perilesional tissue for direct immunofluorescence if routine biopsy is not diagnostic

MANAGEMENT

- Systemic corticosteroids
- Steroid-sparing agents
- Systemic antibiotics, used as anti-inflammatory agents
- Antimalarial agents
- Topical corticosteroids

SPECIFIC THERAPY

- Prednisone 1–2 mg/kg PO QAM
- Hydroxychloroquine 200 mg PO BID
- Steroid-sparing agents
  - Azathioprine 2–3 mg/kg PO QD
  - Dapsone 100–200 mg PO QD
  - Mycophenolate mofetil 1–1.5 g PO BID
  - Cyclophosphamide 100–200 mg PO QD

CAVEATS AND PITFALLS

- If prednisone is to be used for >21 days per course of therapy, obtain baseline chest radiograph, TB skin test & bone mineral density determination.

- Check thiopurine methyltransferase levels before starting azathioprine therapy.
- Check CBC Q2–3 weeks for 10–12 weeks w/ dapsone to detect rare pancytopenia.
  - Obtain baseline G6PD level before dapsone therapy.
- Mycophenolate mofetil is associated w/ fatigue & GI disturbances.

PEMPHIGUS VULGARIS

ALTERNATE DISEASE NAME
- None

HISTORY
- Insidious onset of painful mouth lesions, which often precede other manifestations of disease

PHYSICAL EXAMINATION
- Mucous membrane lesions
  - Ill-defined, irregularly shaped, gingival, buccal or palatine erosions, most commonly in oral cavity
  - Lesions may spread to larynx w/ subsequent hoarseness
  - Other sites of mucous membrane involvement include conjunctiva, esophagus, labia, vagina, cervix, penis, urethra & anus
- Skin lesions
  - Fragile, flaccid vesicle or bulla, arising on normal skin or on an inflammatory base
  - Large erosions w/ lateral spread of blisters
- Vegetating (vegetans) variant
  - Lesions in skin folds evolve into vegetating plaques w/ excessive granulation tissue & crusting
  - Occurs preferentially in intertriginous areas & on scalp or face

DIFFERENTIAL DIAGNOSIS
- Pemphigus foliaceus
- Aphthous stomatitis
- Paraneoplastic pemphigus

- Bullous pemphigoid
- Erythema multiforme
- Herpes simplex virus infection
- Dermatitis herpetiformis
- Hailey-Hailey disease
- Erosive lichen planus

LABORATORY WORK-UP
- Biopsy of fresh lesion for routine histology
- Biopsy of perilesional tissue for direct immunofluorescence if routine biopsy is not diagnostic

MANAGEMENT
- Systemic corticosteroids
- Steroid-sparing agents
- Topical corticosteroids

SPECIFIC THERAPY
- Prednisone 1–2 mg/kg PO QAM
- Steroid-sparing agents
  - Mycophenolate mofetil 1–1.5 g PO BID
  - Azathioprine 2–3 mg/kg PO QD
  - Dapsone 100–200 mg PO QD
  - Cyclophosphamide 100–200 mg PO QD
  - Cyclosporine 3–5 mg/kg PO QD
  - Auranofin 3–6 mg PO QD
  - Intravenous immunoglobulin (IVIg) 2 g IV divided over 3 days every 4–8 weeks

CAVEATS AND PITFALLS
- If prednisone is to be used for >21 days per course of therapy, obtain baseline chest radiograph, TB skin test & bone mineral density determination.
- Mycophenolate mofetil is associated w/ fatigue & GI disturbances.
- Check thiopurine methyltransferase levels before starting azathioprine therapy.
- Check CBC Q2–3 weeks for 10–12 weeks w/ dapsone to detect rare pancytopenia.
  - Obtain baseline G6PD level before dapsone therapy.

PERFORATING FOLLICULITIS

ALTERNATE DISEASE NAME
- Acquired perforating dermatosis
- Acquired perforating dermatitis

HISTORY
- May be associated w/ diabetes mellitus & renal failure
- Chronic, recurrent lesions w/ minimal pruritus & occasional spontaneous remission

PHYSICAL EXAMINATION
- Papules concentrated on hair-bearing portions of extremities & buttocks
- Scaly follicle-based papules, w/ small central keratotic plugs & varying degrees of erythema

DIFFERENTIAL DIAGNOSIS
- Folliculitis
- Elastosis perforans serpiginosa
- Kyrle disease
- Reactive perforating collagenosis
- Perforating granuloma annulare
- Prurigo nodularis
- Acne vulgaris
- Pseudofolliculitis barbae
- Insect bite reaction

LABORATORY WORK-UP
- Lesional biopsy for routine histology

MANAGEMENT
- Topical retinoids

SPECIFIC THERAPY
- Tretinoin 0.025% cream applied QD

CAVEATS AND PITFALLS
- Only fair response to therapy.

PERIORAL DERMATITIS

ALTERNATE DISEASE NAME
- Periorificial dermatitis
- Rosacea-like dermatitis
- Steroid rosacea
- Chronic papulopustular facial dermatitis
- Papulopustular facial dermatitis
- Granulomatous perioral dermatitis

HISTORY
- Often associated w/ use of potent topical corticosteroids on face

PHYSICAL EXAMINATION
- Located mainly in perioral area, but also in nasolabial fold & lateral portions of lower eyelids
- Grouped follicular papules, papulovesicles & papulopustules on an erythematous base
- Lesions may coalesce into plaques

DIFFERENTIAL DIAGNOSIS
- Rosacea
- Seborrheic dermatitis
- Acne vulgaris
- Lupus erythematosus
- Tinea faciei
- Contact dermatitis
- Haber syndrome

LABORATORY WORK-UP
- None

MANAGEMENT
- Discontinue use of topical corticosteroids to face
- Systemic antibiotics used as anti-inflammatory agents

SPECIFIC THERAPY
- Tetracycline 500 mg PO BID for at least 4 weeks
- Doxycycline 100 mg PO BID for at least 4 weeks
- Minocycline 50–100 mg PO BID for at least 4 weeks
- Erythromycin 500 mg PO BID for at least 4 weeks

CAVEATS AND PITFALLS
- Advise about temporary flare of disease after stopping topical corticosteroids & starting systemic antibiotics.

PEUTZ-JEGHERS SYNDROME

ALTERNATE DISEASE NAME
- None

HISTORY
- Gradual increase in asymptomatic pigmented lesions
- Familial clustering

PHYSICAL EXAMINATION
- Macular hyperpigmentation on inner lining of mouth, gums, lips, around mouth, around eyes, fingers or toes & genitalia
- Pigmentation varies in color from bluish black to dark brown to blue; may fade over time
- Dozens to thousands of hamartomatous polyps in stomach & intestines, primarily in small bowel

DIFFERENTIAL DIAGNOSIS
- Familial adenomatous polyposis
- Cowden disease
- Juvenile polyposis
- Carney syndrome
- Cronkhite-Canada syndrome Ruvalcaba-Myhre-Smith
- Turcot syndrome

LABORATORY WORK-UP
- None

MANAGEMENT
- Repeated GI endoscopic examinations
- Surgical removal of polyps suspicious for malignancy

SPECIFIC THERAPY
- None

CAVEATS AND PITFALLS
- None

PIEBALDISM

ALTERNATE DISEASE NAME
- Partial albinism
- Familial white spotting

HISTORY
- Permanently white hair & skin lesions, present from birth

PHYSICAL EXAMINATION
- White area of both hair & skin in central frontal scalp, often in triangular shape
- May affect eyebrow & eyelash hair
- Symmetrical, irregular, hypopigmented macules & patches on face, trunk & extremities
- White lesions may have narrow border of hyperpigmentation or island of pigmentation

DIFFERENTIAL DIAGNOSIS
- Albinism
- Nevus depigmentosus
- Hypomelanosis of Ito
- Waardenburg's syndrome
- Vogt-Koyanagi-Harada syndrome
- Vitiligo
- Chemical leukoderma
- Onchocerciasis
- Pinta
- Leprosy
- Tinea versicolor
- Pityriasis alba

LABORATORY WORK-UP
- None

MANAGEMENT
- Sun protection of white patches

SPECIFIC THERAPY
- None

CAVEATS AND PITFALLS
- None

PIEDRA

ALTERNATE DISEASE NAME
- Black piedra
- White piedra
- Trichosporosis
- Tinea nodosa
- Trichomycosis nodularis

HISTORY
- Occurs mostly in tropical climates
- Increased carriage rate in HIV-positive pts
- May be sexually transmitted
- Caused by 2 superficial fungal pathogens: *Piedraia hortae*, causing black piedra, & *Trichosporon beigelii*, causing white piedra

PHYSICAL EXAMINATION
- Black piedra
  - Firmly adherent, black, firm, oval or elongated papules, composed of a mass of fungus cells
  - Scalp most common site, but also seen in beard & pubic areas
- White piedra
  - Soft, white or light-brown papules loosely adherent to or within the hair shaft
  - Scalp most common site of involvement, but also seen in beard & pubic areas

DIFFERENTIAL DIAGNOSIS
- Pediculosis
- Tinea capitis
- Tinea corporis
- Trichomycosis axillaris
- Axillary granular hyperkeratosis

LABORATORY WORK-UP
- Microscopic exam of hair shaft

MANAGEMENT
- Shave or cut affected hair
- Topical or systemic antifungal agents

SPECIFIC THERAPY
- Black piedra
  - Terbinafine
    - Adults: 250 mg PO QD for 1 month
    - Children weighing >40 kg: 250 mg PO for 1 month; children weighing 20–40 kg: 125 mg PO for 1 month
- White piedra
  - Clotrimazole 1% cream applied BID for 1 month

CAVEATS AND PITFALLS
- None

PIEZOGENIC PAPULE

ALTERNATE DISEASE NAME
- Piezogenic pedal papule
- Painful piezogenic papule

HISTORY
- Usually asymptomatic lesions, which appear during adult life
- More common in overweight people, those w/ flat feet, pts w/ Ehlers-Danlos syndrome & those who spend significant time on their feet

PHYSICAL EXAMINATION
- Flesh-colored papules over medial, posterior & lateral aspects of heels, usually occurring bilaterally
- May temporarily resolve w/ less weight-bearing activity

DIFFERENTIAL DIAGNOSIS
- Wart
- Benign adnexal tumor
- Foreign body granuloma

LABORATORY WORK-UP
- None

MANAGEMENT
- Heel cup in shoe to minimize herniation in symptomatic lesions

SPECIFIC THERAPY
■ See "Management"

CAVEATS AND PITFALLS
■ None

PILAR CYST

ALTERNATE DISEASE NAME
■ Trichilemmal cyst
■ Scalp cyst
■ Wen
■ Keratinous cyst

HISTORY
■ Spontaneously arises at any age, often on scalp

PHYSICAL EXAMINATION
■ Smooth, firm subcutaneous nodule, w/out a punctum

DIFFERENTIAL DIAGNOSIS
■ Epidermoid cyst
■ Pilomatricoma
■ Dermoid cyst
■ Lipoma
■ Organized hematoma

LABORATORY WORK-UP
■ None

MANAGEMENT
■ Surgical excision

SPECIFIC THERAPY
■ See "Management"

CAVEATS AND PITFALLS
■ Surgical removal indicated only for cosmetic reasons or if the lesion becomes inflamed.

PINTA

ALTERNATE DISEASE NAME
- Endemic treponematosis
- Mal de pinto
- Azul
- Carate

HISTORY
- May be transmitted by direct skin or mucous membrane contact
- Pts remain otherwise well

PHYSICAL EXAMINATION
- Initial lesion is a papule that slowly enlarges to become pruritic plaque, often on dorsum of foot & legs
- Lesions become pigmented over time, sometimes becoming copper to slate gray in color
- Late lesions are achromic or hyperpigmented
- Regional lymphadenopathy

DIFFERENTIAL DIAGNOSIS
- Postinflammatory hypopigmentation
- Pityriasis alba
- Yaws
- Leprosy
- Tinea corporis
- Tinea versicolor
- Vitiligo
- Syphilis

LABORATORY WORK-UP
- Dark-field exam of exudate from early lesion
- Serologic test for syphilis

MANAGEMENT
- Systemic antibiotics

SPECIFIC THERAPY
- Penicillin G 2.4 million units IM (over age 10); 1.2 million units IM (<10 years old)
- Penicillin-allergic pts

➤ Tetracycline 500 mg PO QID for 15 days; indicated for pts over age 8 years

➤ Erythromycin 500 mg PO QID for 15 days

CAVEATS AND PITFALLS
■ None

PITTED KERATOLYSIS

ALTERNATE DISEASE NAME
■ Ringed keratolysis
■ Keratoma plantarum sulcatum
■ Keratolysis plantaris sulcatum

HISTORY
■ Occurs in the context of prolonged occlusion, hyperhidrosis & increased skin surface pH on feet

PHYSICAL EXAMINATION
■ Superficial pits, w/ some confluence into plaques
■ Irregular erosions, or sulci, most often on plantar aspects of feet
■ Usually asymptomatic, but sometimes malodor, hyperhidrosis, sliminess & occasional soreness or itching

DIFFERENTIAL DIAGNOSIS
■ Tinea pedis
■ Essential hyperhidrosis
■ Plantar warts
■ Basal cell nevus syndrome
■ Keratolysis exfoliativa
■ Punctate keratoderma
■ Arsenical keratoses

LABORATORY WORK-UP
■ None

MANAGEMENT
■ Topical antibiotics
■ Systemic antibiotics
■ Minimize use of occlusive footwear
■ Reduce foot friction w/ properly fitting shoes

■ Wear absorbent cotton socks & change them frequently

SPECIFIC THERAPY
■ Erythromycin 500 mg PO QID for 10 days
■ Erythromycin 2% solution applied BID for 2–4 weeks

CAVEATS AND PITFALLS
■ None

PITYRIASIS ALBA

ALTERNATE DISEASE NAME
■ Pityriasis simplex
■ Pityriasis sicca faciei

HISTORY
■ Occurs mainly in children, many of whom are atopic

PHYSICAL EXAMINATION
■ Solitary or multiple, red, pink or skin-colored, round or oval, irregular plaques, w/ pityriasiform scale, most often on face, neck & lateral arms

DIFFERENTIAL DIAGNOSIS
■ Tinea corporis
■ Tinea versicolor
■ Sarcoidosis
■ Vitiligo
■ Psoriasis
■ Leprosy
■ Mycosis fungoides
■ Seborrheic dermatitis
■ Nummular eczema

LABORATORY WORK-UP
■ Potassium hydroxide preparation to rule out dermatophyte (superficial fungal) infection

MANAGEMENT
■ Topical corticosteroids
■ Emollients

SPECIFIC THERAPY
- Hydrocortisone 1% cream applied BID

CAVEATS AND PITFALLS
- Judicious sunlight exposure can increase skin pigmentation after topical corticosteroid therapy.

PITYRIASIS LICHENOIDES

ALTERNATE DISEASE NAME
- Pityriasis lichenoides et varioliformis acuta
- Mucha-Habermann disease
- Guttate parapsoriasis
- Pityriasis lichenoides chronica

HISTORY
- Abrupt onset w/ acute variant, sometimes w/ mild constitutional symptoms
- Insidious onset in subacute or chronic form

PHYSICAL EXAMINATION
- Acute variant (Mucha-Habermann disease)
  - Multiple pruritic papules on trunk, buttocks & proximal extremities, evolving to vesicles that rupture & produce hemorrhagic crusts
  - Lesions heal w/ postinflammatory hypo- or hyperpigmentation
- Chronic variant (pityriasis lichenoides chronica)
  - Small erythematous to reddish-brown papules distributed over trunk, buttocks & proximal extremities, w/ fine scale
  - May have polymorphic lesions at different stages of evolution

DIFFERENTIAL DIAGNOSIS
- Acute variant
  - Varicella
  - Vasculitis
  - Insect bite reaction
  - Scabies
  - Dermatitis herpetiformis
  - External trauma

- Chronic variant
  - Pityriasis rosea
  - Tinea corporis
  - Psoriasis
  - Small plaque parapsoriasis
  - Mycosis fungoides
  - Lupus erythematosus
  - Syphilis
  - Viral exanthem

LABORATORY WORK-UP
- Lesional biopsy if diagnosis is in doubt

MANAGEMENT
- Methotrexate
- Systemic antibiotics as anti-inflammatory agents
- Phototherapy
- Topical corticosteroids

SPECIFIC THERAPY
- Acute variant
  - Methotrexate 5–7.5 mg PO weekly
  - Tetracycline 500 mg PO BID
  - Erythromycin 500 mg PO BID
- Chronic variant
  - Phototherapy
  - Fluocinonide 0.05% cream applied BID

CAVEATS AND PITFALLS
- If there are no contraindications, use methotrexate as treatment of choice in acute variant.
- Systemic antibiotics used as anti-inflammatory agents in this disease.

PITYRIASIS ROSEA

ALTERNATE DISEASE NAME
- None

HISTORY
- Often begins w/ solitary lesion (herald patch) a few days before onset of a more generalized eruption

PHYSICAL EXAMINATION
- Multiple, salmon-colored, scaly papules; long axes of lesions oriented in parallel fashion along cleavage lines
- Occurs most commonly on trunk, abdomen, back & proximal upper extremities
- Clears in 6–12 weeks, w/ only rare recurrences

DIFFERENTIAL DIAGNOSIS
- Syphilis
- Pityriasis lichenoides
- Tinea corporis
- Viral exanthem
- Nummular eczema
- Mycosis fungoides
- Lupus erythematosus
- Drug eruption

LABORATORY WORK-UP
- Serologic test to rule out syphilis

MANAGEMENT
- Phototherapy
- Systemic antibiotics

SPECIFIC THERAPY
- Erythromycin 500 mg PO BID for 2 weeks

CAVEATS AND PITFALLS
- If eruption persists for >8–10 weeks, consider pityriasis lichenoides chronica as diagnostic possibility.

PITYRIASIS RUBRA PILARIS

ALTERNATE DISEASE NAME
- None

HISTORY
- May present as seborrheic dermatitis-like eruption
- Subsequent spread from head downward

PHYSICAL EXAMINATION
- Orange-red or salmon-colored scaling plaques w/ sharp borders, which may expand to become whole-body erythroderma, w/ islands of sparing
- Follicular hyperkeratosis on dorsal aspects of proximal phalanges, elbows & wrists
- Palmoplantar hyperkeratosis
- Nails w/ distal yellow-brown discoloration, subungual hyperkeratosis, longitudinal ridging, nail plate thickening & splinter hemorrhages
- Subtypes
  - Type I
    - Most common form
    - Acute onset of erythroderma w/ islands of sparing, palmoplantar keratoderma & follicular hyperkeratosis
    - 80% of pts have remission in about 3 years
  - Type II
    - Ichthyosiform lesions w/ areas of eczematous changes
    - Alopecia
    - Very long duration of disease
  - Type III is very similar to type I, but onset is within the first 2 years of life
  - Type IV appears in prepubertal children w/ sharply demarcated areas of follicular hyperkeratosis & erythema of knees & elbows, w/out progression
  - Type V
    - Most familial cases belong to this group
    - Early onset, chronic course
    - Prominent follicular hyperkeratosis; scleroderma-like changes on palms & soles, w/ occasional erythema
  - Type VI
    - HIV-associated
    - Cystic & pustular acneiform lesions
    - Resistant to standard treatments but sometimes responds to antiretroviral therapies

DIFFERENTIAL DIAGNOSIS
- Psoriasis
- Other causes of exfoliative erythroderma, including T-cell lymphoma, drug eruption, atopic dermatitis, pemphigus foliaceus, seborrheic dermatitis
- Erythroderma variabilis

LABORATORY WORK-UP
- Skin biopsy if diagnosis is in doubt

MANAGEMENT
- Systemic anti-inflammatory agents

SPECIFIC THERAPY
- Methotrexate 10–25 mg PO weekly
- Cyclosporine 3–5 mg/kg PO QD
- Acitretin 50–75 mg PO QD
- Thioguanine 120–160 mg PO 2 or 3 times weekly

CAVEATS AND PITFALLS
- Check for possible liver dysfunction while on methotrexate.
- Systemic retinoids are contraindicated in women of child-bearing potential.
- Check thiopurine methyltransferase levels before starting thioguanine therapy.

POIKILODERMA OF CIVATTE

ALTERNATE DISEASE NAME
- Berkshire neck

HISTORY
- Occurs after chronic sun exposure, mostly in fair-skinned people

PHYSICAL EXAMINATION
- Reddish-brown reticulate pigmentation w/ atrophy & telangiectasia
- Occurs in symmetrical plaques on sides of neck

DIFFERENTIAL DIAGNOSIS
- Lupus erythematosus
- Dermatomyositis
- Berloque dermatitis
- Poikiloderma atrophicans vasculare
- Rothmund-Thomson syndrome
- Bloom syndrome
- Riehl's melanosis

LABORATORY WORK-UP
- None

MANAGEMENT
- Intense pulse light (IPL) therapy
- Flashlamp-pumped pulsed-dye laser (FPDL, 585 nm)
- Potassium-titanyl-phosphate (KTP) laser

SPECIFIC THERAPY
- See "Management"

CAVEATS AND PITFALLS
- None

POLYARTERITIS NODOSA

ALTERNATE DISEASE NAME
- Periarteritis nodosa

HISTORY
- Constitutional signs & symptoms include fever, weight loss, myalgias & abdominal pain
- Associated w/ viral hepatitis in some pts

PHYSICAL EXAMINATION
- Cutaneous findings
  - Palpable purpura
  - Cutaneous infarctions w/ ulceration
  - Discontinuous livedo reticularis (retiform purpura)
  - Ischemic changes of distal digits
  - Subcutaneous nodules

■ Systemic disease includes mesenteric thrombosis & ischemia, renal vascular nephropathy, sensory & motor neuropathies, mononeuritis multiplex, coronary arteritis, tachycardia & retinal vasculitis

DIFFERENTIAL DIAGNOSIS
■ Microscopic polyangiitis
■ Septicemia
■ Infective endocarditis
■ Sjögren syndrome
■ Cryoglobulinemia
■ Lupus erythematosus
■ Malignancy
■ Atherosclerosis
■ Rheumatoid arthritis

LABORATORY WORK-UP
■ Hepatitis screen
■ ESR, C-reactive protein
■ Chemistry screen
■ Tissue biopsy, such as skin, sural nerve, testes or skeletal muscle, depending on site of clinical involvement
■ Visceral angiogram if involved tissue is not accessible by less invasive means

MANAGEMENT
■ Systemic corticosteroids
■ Steroid-sparing agents

SPECIFIC THERAPY
■ Prednisone 1–2 mg/kg PO QAM
■ Cyclophosphamide 100–200 mg PO QD
■ Cyclosporine 3–5 mg/kg PO QD

CAVEATS AND PITFALLS
■ If prednisone is to be used for >21 days per course of therapy, obtain baseline chest radiograph, TB skin test & bone mineral density determination.
■ Check renal status & blood pressure regularly while on cyclosporine.

POLYMORPHOUS LIGHT ERUPTION

ALTERNATE DISEASE NAME
- Polymorphic light eruption

HISTORY
- Directly related to sunlight exposure
- Usual onset is in early spring or immediately after sunny vacation, w/ improvement as sunny season continues
- Eruption appears within hours to days of exposure & subsides over the next 1–7 days w/out scarring

PHYSICAL EXAMINATION
- Pruritic papules, plaques, papulovesicles & erythema multiforme-like lesions, often combined in the same pt
- Small papules may coalesce to form eczematous plaques
- Sun-exposed skin, especially that normally covered in winter, is most commonly affected
- Autosensitization may lead to generalized involvement
- Cheilitis occurs mainly in Native American children w/ a combined polymorphous light & atopic dermatitis-like syndrome (actinic prurigo)

DIFFERENTIAL DIAGNOSIS
- Lupus erythematosus
- Solar urticaria
- Erythropoietic protoporphyria
- Drug-induced photosensitivity
- Actinic dermatitis
- Hydroa vacciniforme

LABORATORY WORK-UP
- Tests to rule out other diseases
  - ANA
  - Ro/SSA
  - 24-hour urine uroporphyrin & coproporphyrin levels
  - Skin biopsy

MANAGEMENT
- Prophylactic phototherapy before onset of sunny season

- Antimalarial agents
- Systemic carotenoids
- Topical corticosteroids
- Systemic corticosteroids only for short-term use in severe disease

SPECIFIC THERAPY
- Hydroxychloroquine 200 mg PO BID
- Thalidomide 100–300 mg PO QD
- Beta-carotene 120–300 mg PO per day
- Fluocinonide 0.05% cream applied BID
- Prednisone 1 mg/kg PO QAM for a maximum of 3 weeks

CAVEATS AND PITFALLS
- Settle on this diagnosis only after ruling out lupus erythematosus.
- Check for retinal toxicity w/ hydroxychloroquine every 6 months.
- Thalidomide is contraindicated in women of child-bearing potential; also advise about possible peripheral neuropathy associated w/ this drug.

POROKERATOSIS

ALTERNATE DISEASE NAME
- Porokeratosis of Mibelli
- Disseminated superficial actinic porokeratosis (DSAP)
- Porokeratosis palmaris et plantaris disseminata
- Linear porokeratosis
- Punctate porokeratosis
- Hyperkeratosis eccentrica
- Hyperkeratosis figurata centrifuga atrophicans

HISTORY
- Insidious onset of asymptomatic lesions
- Familial clustering of disseminated superficial actinic porokeratosis variant

PHYSICAL EXAMINATION
- Porokeratosis of Mibelli: slowly expanding, irregularly shaped plaque w/ a raised, thready border, which may be slightly

hypopigmented or hyperpigmented, minimally scaly, hairless, slightly atrophic & anhidrotic
- Disseminated superficial actinic porokeratosis: multiple, small, indistinct, light-brown papules w/ a threadlike border, on extensor surface of upper & lower extremities
- Linear porokeratosis: grouped, linear, annular papules & plaques w/ a raised peripheral ridge on extremity, trunk and/or head & neck area, often in a dermatomal pattern

DIFFERENTIAL DIAGNOSIS
- Actinic keratosis
- Elastosis perforans serpiginosa
- Granuloma annulare
- Superficial basal cell carcinoma
- Annular lichen planus
- Squamous cell carcinoma
- Flat warts

LABORATORY WORK-UP
- Skin biopsy to confirm diagnosis

MANAGEMENT
- Destructive modalities such as liquid nitrogen cryotherapy, electrodesiccation & curettage & dermabrasion
- Topical fluorouracil
- Topical immune modulators
- Topical calcipotriene
- Systemic retinoids

SPECIFIC THERAPY
- Fluorouracil 0.5–5% cream applied 1 or 2 times daily for 4–8 weeks
- Imiquimod 5% cream applied 3 times weekly for 4–8 weeks
- Calcipotriene 0.005% ointment applied BID for 4–8 weeks
- Isotretinoin 1 mg/kg PO QD for 4–5 months

CAVEATS AND PITFALLS
- Multiple treatment courses may be needed to clear eruption completely.
- Systemic retinoids are contraindicated in women of childbearing potential.

PORPHYRIA CUTANEA TARDA

ALTERNATE DISEASE NAME
- Hepatic porphyria

HISTORY
- Associated w/ liver diseases such as viral hepatitis, hepatoma & chronic alcoholism
- Flares after sun exposure & mechanical trauma

PHYSICAL EXAMINATION
- Erosions & bullae, most commonly on dorsal hands, forearms & face
- Healing of erosions & blisters leaves scars, milia & dyspigmentation
- Hypertrichosis, mostly over temporal & malar facial areas
- Melasma-like hyperpigmentation of face
- Red suffusion of central face, neck, upper chest & shoulder
- Scarring alopecia of scalp
- Photo-onycholysis
- Scleroderma-like papules on trunk & extremities

DIFFERENTIAL DIAGNOSIS
- Pseudoporphyria
- Other forms of porphyria
- Bullous pemphigoid
- Epidermolysis bullosa acquisita
- Bullous diabeticorum
- Bullous lupus erythematosus
- Polymorphous light eruption

LABORATORY WORK-UP
- 24-hour uroporphyrin & coproporphyrin levels
- Liver function studies
- Serum iron & ferritin levels

MANAGEMENT
- Therapeutic phlebotomy, 1 unit every 2–3 weeks until clinical response or until hemoglobin falls below 10.5–11 g
- Antimalarial agents

SPECIFIC THERAPY
- Hydroxychloroquine 200 mg PO TIW; increase dose slowly over several months until a dose of 200 mg QD is reached; monitor for hepatic dysfunction

CAVEATS AND PITFALLS
- Rapid increases in hydroxychloroquine dosage can produce acute liver toxicity.
- Check for retinal toxicity w/ hydroxychloroquine every 6 months.

POSTINFLAMMATORY HYPERPIGMENTATION

ALTERNATE DISEASE NAME
- Postinflammatory hypermelanosis
- Melanotic hyperpigmentation

HISTORY
- Occurs after inflammatory process
- More common in those w/ dark skin

PHYSICAL EXAMINATION
- Irregular, light-brown to black macules and/or patches at sites of prior inflammation

DIFFERENTIAL DIAGNOSIS
- Melasma
- Tinea versicolor
- Acanthosis nigricans
- Lichen planus
- Lupus erythematosus
- Nevoid hypermelanosis
- Amyloidosis
- Ashy dermatosis

LABORATORY WORK-UP
- None

MANAGEMENT
- Bleaching agents
- Sunscreens

SPECIFIC THERAPY
- Hydroquinone 4% cream applied BID for at least 3 months
- Azelaic acid 15–20% applied BID for at least 3 months

CAVEATS AND PITFALLS
- Marginal improvement w/ therapies.

PROGRESSIVE SYSTEMIC SCLEROSIS

ALTERNATE DISEASE NAME
- Systemic sclerosis
- Scleroderma
- Systemic connective tissue disease
- Diffuse systemic sclerosis

HISTORY
- Many different presentations, including pruritus, Raynaud phenomenon, dyspnea, arthralgias, weakness & palpitations

PHYSICAL EXAMINATION
- Skin
  - Areas of hyperpigmentation alternating w/ hypopigmentation
  - Tanned skin persisting long after sun exposure
  - Telangiectasias on face, neck & periungual area
  - Edematous skin of hands preceding sclerotic stage, where skin is tight & shiny, w/ loss of hair, decreased sweating & loss of ability to make a skin fold, beginning on fingers
  - Calcinosis on extremities
  - Reduced oral aperture (microstomia) from perioral involvement
- Vascular changes
  - Raynaud phenomenon triggered by cold, smoking or emotional stress
  - Infarction & dry gangrene, sometimes resulting from severe vasospasm
- Ears, nose & throat
  - Xerostomia & xerophthalmia
- Musculoskeletal system
  - Arthralgias & morning stiffness sometimes

➤ Acroosteolysis (ie., resorption or dissolution of distal end of phalanx)
➤ Flexion contractures
■ Neurologic system
➤ Trigeminal neuralgia
➤ Carpal tunnel symptoms
■ Respiratory system
➤ Dry rales, indicating fibrosis
➤ Esophageal sphincter incompetence
■ GI system
➤ Reflux esophagitis
➤ Barrett metaplasia
➤ Candidiasis
➤ Watermelon stomach or gastric vascular antral ectasia
➤ Primary biliary cirrhosis
➤ Malabsorption
➤ Atrophy of smooth muscle & fibrotic changes leading to decreased peristalsis throughout GI tract
■ Renal failure
■ Cardiac
➤ Pericardial effusions w/ cor pulmonale
➤ Conduction abnormalities
➤ Infiltrative cardiomyopathy

DIFFERENTIAL DIAGNOSIS
■ Morphea
■ Linear scleroderma
■ Eosinophilia-myalgia syndrome
■ Bleomycin-induced scleroderma
■ Toxic oil syndrome
■ Porphyria cutanea tarda
■ Digital sclerosis of diabetes mellitus
■ Radiation exposure
■ Intestinal obstruction from other causes
■ Infiltrative cardiomyopathy from other causes
■ Chronic graft-versus-host disease

LABORATORY WORK-UP
■ Renal & cardiac function studies

- Pulmonary function studies if there are symptoms of decreased function
- GI motility studies as per clinical findings

MANAGEMENT
- D-penicillamine
- Methotrexate
- Active physical therapy

SPECIFIC THERAPY
- D-penicillamine 250–1,500 mg per day PO divided into 2 or 3 doses
- Methotrexate 7.5–25 mg PO once weekly

CAVEATS AND PITFALLS
- Modest benefits from medical therapies.
- Treatment of choice is active physical therapy.

PRURIGO OF PREGNANCY

ALTERNATE DISEASE NAME
- Pruritus of pregnancy
- Prurigo gestationis
- Early-onset prurigo of pregnancy
- Papular dermatitis of pregnancy
- Pruritic folliculitis of pregnancy

HISTORY
- Usually occurs in last trimester of pregnancy
- May have jaundice w/ cholestasis

PHYSICAL EXAMINATION
- Generalized pruritus, w/ papules produced by scratching

DIFFERENTIAL DIAGNOSIS
- Pruritic urticarial papules & plaques of pregnancy
- Pemphigoid gestationis (herpes gestationis)
- Scabies
- Insect bite reaction
- Impetigo herpetiformis

LABORATORY WORK-UP
- None

MANAGEMENT
- Topical corticosteroids

SPECIFIC THERAPY
- Triamcinolone 0.1% cream applied BID

CAVEATS AND PITFALLS
- Resolves promptly after parturition.

PRURITIC URTICARIAL PAPULES AND PLAQUES OF PREGNANCY

ALTERNATE DISEASE NAME
- PUPPP
- Polymorphic eruption of pregnancy
- Toxemic erythema of pregnancy
- Toxemic rash of pregnancy
- Late-onset prurigo of pregnancy

HISTORY
- Typically arises in third trimester, particularly in first pregnancy
- No adverse fetal effects

PHYSICAL EXAMINATION
- Erythematous urticarial papules & plaques of trunk & extremities & in striae
- Periumbilical area spared

DIFFERENTIAL DIAGNOSIS
- Urticaria
- Erythema multiforme
- Prurigo gestationis
- Viral exanthem
- Drug eruption
- Cholestasis of pregnancy
- Impetigo herpetiformis
- Herpes gestationis
- Papular dermatitis of pregnancy

LABORATORY WORK-UP
- None

MANAGEMENT
- Topical corticosteroids
- Systemic corticosteroids only for severe flares

SPECIFIC THERAPY
- Fluocinonide 0.05% cream applied BID
- Prednisone 1 mg/kg PO QAM for 7–14 days

CAVEATS AND PITFALLS
- Resolves within weeks of parturition, but may recur in subsequent pregnancies.

PSEUDOFOLLICULITIS BARBAE

ALTERNATE DISEASE NAME
- Pseudofolliculitis of the beard
- Shaving bumps
- Razor bumps
- Pili incarnati
- Folliculitis barbae traumatica

HISTORY
- Occurs in those w/ curly or kinky hair

PHYSICAL EXAMINATION
- Flesh-colored or erythematous papule w/ central hair shaft in shaved areas adjacent to follicular ostia
- Pustules & abscess formation from secondary infection
- Postinflammatory hyperpigmentation
- Scarring & keloid formation possible

DIFFERENTIAL DIAGNOSIS
- Folliculitis
- Acne vulgaris
- Tinea barbae
- Acne keloidalis
- Rosacea
- Sarcoidosis
- Granuloma annulare

LABORATORY WORK-UP
- None

MANAGEMENT
- Grow a beard, if possible
- Shaving techniques to minimize trauma
  - Discontinue shaving for at least 3–4 weeks
  - Cleanse beard w/ face cloth, wet sponge, or soft-bristled toothbrush w/ a mild soap for several minutes before shaving
  - Use foil-guarded safety razor
  - Electric razors are acceptable if used properly: 3-headed, rotary electric razor w/ heads slightly off skin surface; shave in a slow circular motion
  - Chemical depilatories
- Laser destruction of hair follicles

SPECIFIC THERAPY
- See "Management"

CAVEATS AND PITFALLS
- If beard growing is not practical, shave daily to avoid ingrowing hairs.

PSEUDOPELADE

ALTERNATE DISEASE NAME
- Pseudopelade of Brocq
- Brocq pseudopelade

HISTORY
- Slowly progressive hair loss from scalp
- No associated signs & symptoms

PHYSICAL EXAMINATION
- Randomly distributed, irregularly shaped areas of scarring alopecia of scalp
- May have hypopigmentation & slight atrophy
- Few hairs may remain in otherwise completely bald & scarred plaque
- No clinical evidence of inflammation

DIFFERENTIAL DIAGNOSIS
- Alopecia areata
- Post-traumatic alopecia
- Folliculitis decalvans
- Androgenetic alopecia
- Lupus erythematosus
- Lichen planus
- Follicular degeneration syndrome
- Lichen sclerosus

LABORATORY WORK-UP
- Scalp biopsy

MANAGEMENT
- No effective therapy

SPECIFIC THERAPY
- None

CAVEATS AND PITFALLS
- None

PSEUDOXANTHOMA ELASTICUM

ALTERNATE DISEASE NAME
- Systematized elastorrhexis
- Grönblad-Strandberg syndrome

HISTORY
- Usually first noted on lateral neck as asymptomatic skin change
- May have accelerated coronary artery disease causing angina pectoris & subsequent myocardial infarction
- Associated GI hemorrhage, usually gastric in origin
- May develop hemorrhage in urinary tract or cerebrovascular system

PHYSICAL EXAMINATION
- Symmetric, small, yellow papules, coalescing into plaques in a linear pattern, giving affected skin "plucked chicken" appearance

- Occurs on lateral neck, antecubital fossae, axillae, popliteal fossae, inguinal & periumbilical areas
- In later stages may involve oral, vaginal & rectal mucosa
- Skin may become soft, lax & wrinkled & hang in folds
- May have coexistent elastosis perforans serpiginosa
- Ocular findings include bilaterally symmetric angioid streaks of retina, retinal hemorrhages; progressive loss of central vision

DIFFERENTIAL DIAGNOSIS
- Actinic damage to lateral neck
- Marfan syndrome
- Ehlers-Danlos syndrome
- Buschke-Ollendorff syndrome
- Localized acquired cutaneous pseudoxanthoma elasticum
- Penicillamine side effect

LABORATORY WORK-UP
- Skin biopsy

MANAGEMENT
- Surgical correction of lax skin
- Diet & exercise to minimize risks associated w/ cardiovascular disease

SPECIFIC THERAPY
- See "Management"

CAVEATS AND PITFALLS
- None

PSORIASIS

ALTERNATE DISEASE NAME
- None

HISTORY
- Familial clustering
- May first arise after streptococcal infection, especially in children
- Associated arthritis in 5% of pts

PHYSICAL EXAMINATION
- Plaque variant
  - Sharply demarcated, red papules & plaques, w/ silvery-white scale, most often located on scalp, trunk & limbs, w/ predilection for extensor surfaces such as elbows & knees
  - Tendency toward bilateral symmetry
  - Occurrence of lesions in traumatized skin (Koebner phenomenon)
  - Lesions may be encircled by a paler peripheral zone (Woronoff ring)
  - Nails w/ pitting, onycholysis, subungual hyperkeratosis, irregular & brown nail bed discoloration (oil-drop sign)
- Pustular variant
  - May first appear after withdrawal of systemic corticosteroids
  - Pt may be systemically ill w/ fever, leukocytosis, generalized or patchy erythema, studded w/ pustules in annular or random configuration
- Guttate variant
  - May follow infection, most commonly streptococcal
  - Multiple, discrete, salmon pink, scaly
  - Drop-like papules, beginning on trunk & proximal extremities & spreading to face, ears & scalp
  - Sparing of palms & soles
- Acrodermatitis continua of Hallopeau variant
  - Pustules on distal fingers & on toes
  - Lesions under nail plates w/ nail plate shedding

DIFFERENTIAL DIAGNOSIS
- Plaque & guttate variants
  - Seborrheic dermatitis
  - Tinea corporis
  - Lupus erythematosus
  - Pityriasis rosea
  - Pityriasis rubra pilaris
  - Syphilis
  - Lichen planus
  - Parapsoriasis
  - Pityriasis lichenoides

- ➤ Cutaneous T-cell lymphoma
- ➤ Nummular eczema
- ■ Pustular variant
  - ➤ Subcorneal pustular dermatosis
  - ➤ Acute generalized exanthematous pustulosis
  - ➤ Septicemia
  - ➤ Infected generalized atopic and/or seborrheic dermatitis
  - ➤ Dyshidrotic eczema
  - ➤ Contact dermatitis
  - ➤ Autosensitization reaction
  - ➤ Vesicular dermatophyte infection

LABORATORY WORK-UP
- ■ Skin biopsy only if diagnosis is in doubt

MANAGEMENT
- ■ Ultraviolet light therapy
- ■ Systemic therapies
  - ➤ Methotrexate
  - ➤ Thioguanine
  - ➤ Cyclosporine
  - ➤ Acitretin
  - ➤ Mycophenolate mofetil
  - ➤ Biologic agents
- ■ Topical therapies
  - ➤ Topical corticosteroids
  - ➤ Coal tar gel
  - ➤ Anthralin
  - ➤ Calcipotriene
  - ➤ Tazarotene
  - ➤ Antiseborrheic shampoos

SPECIFIC THERAPY
- ■ Systemic therapy
  - ➤ Methotrexate 5–25 mg PO Q7days
  - ➤ Thioguanine 120–160 mg PO 2 or 3 times weekly
  - ➤ Cyclosporine 3–5 mg/kg PO QD
  - ➤ Acitretin 25–50 mg PO QD
  - ➤ Mycophenolate mofetil 1.5–3 g PO QD
  - ➤ Alefacept 7.5 mg IM weekly for 12 weeks

- ➤ Etanercept 50 mg SQ BIW for 3 months; then 50 mg SQ 1/wk
- ➤ Efalizumab 1 mg/kg sub Q once weekly
- Topical therapy
  - ➤ Clobetasol 0.05% cream applied BID
  - ➤ Coal tar gel applied QD
  - ➤ Anthralin 0.1%-1% applied for 15–30 minutes QD
  - ➤ Calcipotriene 0.005% cream applied QD
  - ➤ Tazarotene 0.3–0.1% cream applied QD
  - ➤ Antiseborrheic shampoos

CAVEATS AND PITFALLS
- Topical therapies are of only very limited utility in generalized disease.
- Avoid systemic corticosteroids, which may destabilize the disease.
- Liver biopsy needed after $\tilde{2}$ g total dose of methotrexate.
- Mycophenolate mofetil associated w/ fatigue & GI disturbances.
- Check for renal impairment & increased blood pressure w/ cyclosporine therapy.
- Biologic agents are very expensive.

PYODERMA GANGRENOSUM

ALTERNATE DISEASE NAME
- None

HISTORY
- Sudden onset of small papule or pustule that rapidly enlarges & becomes ulcerated
- May begin at site of mild skin trauma
- Associated w/ inflammatory bowel disease, polyarthritis & myelogenous leukemia or monoclonal gammopathy

PHYSICAL EXAMINATION
- Classic variety
  - ➤ Small, red papule or pustule evolving rapidly into deep ulceration, w/ violaceous undermined border
  - ➤ Occurs most commonly on legs but may be seen on any skin surface, including around stoma sites (peristomal pyoderma gangrenosum)

> Intraoral ulcerated plaques (pyostomatitis vegetans) occur mainly in pts w/ inflammatory bowel disease
- Atypical variety
  > Vesiculopustular component only at border, w/ erosion or superficial ulceration
  > Occurs most commonly on dorsal aspect of hands, extensor surface of forearms or face
  > Pyoderma vegetans variety: crusted, hyperplastic plaques w/out deep ulceration, similar to that seen in pyostomatitis vegetans

DIFFERENTIAL DIAGNOSIS
- Vasculitis
- Acute febrile neutrophilic dermatosis
- Spider bite reaction
- Trauma
- Wegener's granulomatosis
- Squamous cell carcinoma
- Sporotrichosis
- Orf
- Milker's nodule
- Herpes simplex virus infection (particularly in immunosuppressed pt)
- Antiphospholipid antibody syndrome
- Anthrax
- Vascular insufficiency
- North American blastomycosis ulceration, including factitial disease
- Tuberculosis
- Tertiary syphilis

LABORATORY WORK-UP
- Work-up for underlying causes if there are localizing signs & symptoms
- Biopsy of early lesion

MANAGEMENT
- Prednisone
- Corticosteroid-sparing agents

SPECIFIC THERAPY
- Prednisone 1–2 mg/kg PO QAM
- Corticosteroid-sparing agents
  - Azathioprine 2–3 mg PO QD
  - Dapsone 50–200 mg PO QD
  - Cyclophosphamide 100–200 mg PO QD
  - Mycophenolate mofetil 2–3 g PO QD
  - Cyclosporine 3–5 mg/kg PO QD

CAVEATS AND PITFALLS
- If prednisone is to be used for >21 days per course of therapy, obtain baseline chest radiograph, TB skin test & bone mineral density determination.
- Check thiopurine methyltransferase levels before starting azathioprine therapy.
- Check CBC Q2–3 weeks for 10–12 weeks w/ dapsone to detect rare pancytopenia.
  - Obtain baseline G6PD level before dapsone therapy.
- Mycophenolate mofetil associated w/ fatigue & GI disturbances.
- Check for renal impairment & increased blood pressure w/ cyclosporine therapy.

PYOGENIC GRANULOMA

ALTERNATE DISEASE NAME
- Lobular capillary hemangioma
- Granuloma pyogenicum
- Granuloma telangiectaticum

HISTORY
- May occur after minor local skin trauma or during pregnancy
- Bleeding of lesion w/ minimal manipulation

PHYSICAL EXAMINATION
- Rapidly enlarging, bright red, friable, polypoid papule or nodule, which erodes or ulcerates
- Occurs most commonly on gingiva, lips, nasal mucosa, face & distal extremities

- May develop multiple recurrent lesions after prior attempts at removal
- When occurring in pregnancy, found along the maxillary intraoral mucosal surface, but any intraoral, perioral & extraoral tissue may be involved

DIFFERENTIAL DIAGNOSIS
- Melanoma
- Capillary hemangioma
- Excess granulation tissue
- Squamous cell carcinoma
- Kaposi's sarcoma
- Atypical fibroxanthoma
- Glomus tumor
- Angioendothelioma
- Angiolymphoid hyperplasia
- Angiosarcoma
- Hemangioendothelioma
- Intravascular angiomatosis
- Tufted hemangioma

LABORATORY WORK-UP
- Lesional biopsy

MANAGEMENT
- Surgical excision
- Destruction by electrodesiccation & curettage

SPECIFIC THERAPY
- See "Management"

CAVEATS AND PITFALLS
- Lesion may recur if incompletely removed.
- Always submit biopsy specimen to rule out melanoma.

RAYNAUD'S DISEASE

ALTERNATE DISEASE NAME
- Raynaud's syndrome
- Raynaud disease

- Raynaud syndrome
- Primary Raynaud's

HISTORY
- Familial clustering
- Associated w/ frequent use of vibrating tools such as jackhammers & sanders
- Associated w/ industrial exposure to polyvinyl chloride

PHYSICAL EXAMINATION
- Paroxysmal color changes: white, blue & red; color changes are usually in order noted, which are completely reversible
- Affected site may change colors at least twice during an episode
- Rare extreme ischemia may result in necrosis & digital ulceration

DIFFERENTIAL DIAGNOSIS
- Raynaud's phenomenon from underlying cause, such as scleroderma, lupus erythematosus, dermatomyositis, rheumatoid arthritis, viral hepatitis or neoplastic disease
- Chilblains
- Frostbite
- Buerger disease
- Paroxysmal nocturnal hemoglobinuria
- Peripheral arterial occlusive disease
- Acrocyanosis
- Carpal tunnel syndrome
- Thoracic outlet syndrome

LABORATORY WORK-UP
- CBC, serum chemistry profile
- Work-up for lupus erythematosus, scleroderma, if clinically indicated

MANAGEMENT
- Minimize cold exposure
- Calcium channel blockers

SPECIFIC THERAPY
- Nifedipine 30–60 mg PO daily

CAVEATS AND PITFALLS
- None

REACTIVE PERFORATING COLLAGENOSIS

ALTERNATE DISEASE NAME
- Acquired perforating disease
- Acquired reactive perforating dermatosis
- Collagenoma perforant verruciforme

HISTORY
- Familial clustering
- Lesions occur at sites of minor trauma

PHYSICAL EXAMINATION
- Flesh-colored, dome-shaped papules w/ a central keratotic plug, most commonly found on extensor surfaces of limbs & dorsa of hands
- May have linear distribution (Koebner phenomenon)
- Scarring occurs after healing

DIFFERENTIAL DIAGNOSIS
- Kyrle's disease
- Perforating folliculitis
- Elastosis perforans serpiginosa
- Prurigo nodularis
- Ferguson-Smith type of multiple keratoacanthoma

LABORATORY WORK-UP
- Lesional biopsy

MANAGEMENT
- Topical retinoids
- Systemic retinoids
- Phototherapy

SPECIFIC THERAPY
- Tretinoin 0.025% cream applied QD
- Adapalene 0.1% gel applied QD
- Isotretinoin 0.5–1 mg/kg PO QD for 4–6 months

CAVEATS AND PITFALLS
- Only fair response to therapy.
- Systemic retinoids contraindicated in pregnant women.

REITER SYNDROME

ALTERNATE DISEASE NAME
- Reiter disease
- Fiessinger-Leroy-Reiter syndrome
- Fiessinger-Leroy syndrome

HISTORY
- Diarrhea & dysenteric syndrome or symptoms of urethritis prior to other findings
- Common syndrome in pts w/ HIV disease

PHYSICAL EXAMINATION
- Circular or gyrate white plaques expanding centrifugally over glans penis (balanitis circinata)
- Conjunctivitis w/ intense red, velvet-like, conjunctival injection
- Joint symptoms resembling rheumatoid arthritis, but asymmetric & often involving single joint
- Psoriasiform cutaneous lesions, w/ palms & soles most commonly involved w/ keratotic papules, plaques & pustules
- Keratoderma blenorrhagica, w/ painful, keratotic papules & plaques & pustules, w/ painful & erosive lesions in tips of fingers & toes
- Nail dystrophy
- Red macules & plaques, w/ diffuse erythema, erosions & bleeding on oral & pharyngeal mucosa
- Circinate lesions on tongue resembling geographic tongue

DIFFERENTIAL DIAGNOSIS
- Psoriasis
- Pityriasis rubra pilaris
- Lichen planus
- Lupus erythematosus
- Dermatomyositis
- Behçet's disease
- Arthritis associated w/ gonococcal disease
- Rheumatoid arthritis
- Septic arthritis
- Mycosis fungoides

- Subcorneal pustulosis of Sneddon-Wilkinson
- Atopic dermatitis
- Acute exanthematous pustulosis
- Other causes of erythroderma

LABORATORY WORK-UP
- None

MANAGEMENT
- Ultraviolet light therapy
- Systemic therapies
- Methotrexate
- Thioguanine
- Cyclosporine
- Acitretin
- Mycophenolate mofetil
- Topical therapies
- Topical corticosteroids
- Coal tar gel
- Anthralin
- Calcipotriene
- Tazarotene
- Antiseborrheic shampoos

SPECIFIC THERAPY
- Systemic therapy
  - Methotrexate 5–25 mg PO Q 7days
  - Thioguanine 120–160 mg PO 2 or 3 times weekly
  - Cyclosporine 3–5 mg/kg PO QD
  - Acitretin 25–75 mg PO QD
  - Mycophenolate mofetil 1.5–3 g PO QD
  - Topical therapy
  - Clobetasol 0.05% cream applied BID
  - Coal tar gel applied QD
  - Anthralin 0.1%-1% applied for 15–30 minutes QD
  - Calcipotriene 0.005% cream applied QD
  - Tazarotene 0.3–0.1% cream applied QD
  - Antiseborrheic shampoos used QD

CAVEATS AND PITFALLS
- Topical therapies are of only very limited utility in generalized disease.

- Avoid systemic corticosteroids, which may destabilize the disease.
- Liver biopsy needed after ~2 g total dose of methotrexate.
- Mycophenolate mofetil associated w/ fatigue & GI disturbances.
- Check for renal impairment & increased blood pressure w/ cyclosporine therapy.

RELAPSING POLYCHONDRITIS

ALTERNATE DISEASE NAME
- Polychondropathy
- Systemic chondromalacia
- Chronic atrophic polychondritis

HISTORY
- May have one or more of the following presenting signs & symptoms: constitutional symptoms, arthritis, sudden ear pain, dysphagia, decreased visual acuity & chest pain

PHYSICAL EXAMINATION
- Erythema & edema overlying inflamed cartilaginous structures
- Vasculitis of skin & other organs
- Sudden onset of unilateral or bilateral auricle pain, swelling & redness, sparing lobules
- Nonerosive, seronegative inflammatory polyarthritis
- Acute nasal chondritis w/ pain & feeling of fullness over nasal bridge
- Episodic inflammation of uveal tract, conjunctivae, sclerae & cornea

DIFFERENTIAL DIAGNOSIS
- Cellulitis
- Polyarteritis nodosa
- Chondrodermatitis nodularis helicis
- Rheumatoid arthritis
- Cogan syndrome
- Infectious perichondritis
- MAGIC syndrome
- Trauma w/ auricular calcification

- Syphilis
- Chronic external otitis

LABORATORY WORK-UP
- None

MANAGEMENT
- Systemic corticosteroids
- Steroid-sparing agents

SPECIFIC THERAPY
- Prednisone 1–2 mg/kg PO QAM
- Corticosteroid-sparing agents
- Azathioprine 2–3 mg/kg PO QD
- Dapsone 100–200 mg PO QD
- Cyclophosphamide 100–200 mg PO QD
- Mycophenolate mofetil 1–1.5 g PO BID
- Cyclosporine 3–5 mg/kg PO QD

CAVEATS AND PITFALLS
- If prednisone is to be used for >21 days per course of therapy, obtain baseline chest radiograph, TB skin test & bone mineral density determination.
- Check thiopurine methyl transferase levels before starting azathioprine therapy.
- Check CBC Q2–3 weeks for 10–12 weeks w/ dapsone to detect rare pancytopenia.
- Obtain baseline G6PD level before dapsone therapy.
- Mycophenolate mofetil associated w/ fatigue & GI disturbances
- Check for renal impairment & increased blood pressure w/ cyclosporine therapy.

RETICULAR ERYTHEMATOUS MUCINOSIS

ALTERNATE DISEASE NAME
- REM syndrome
- Round cell erythematosus

HISTORY
- Associated w/ sun exposure

PHYSICAL EXAMINATION
- Asymptomatic or slightly pruritic, persistent, erythematous infiltrated papules
- Lesions isolated or coalesce into plaques, in midline of back or chest

DIFFERENTIAL DIAGNOSIS
- Lupus erythematosus
- Scleredema
- Scleromyxedema
- Papular mucinosis
- Generalized myxedema
- Pretibial myxedema
- Focal mucinosis
- Cutaneous mucinosis of infancy
- Nevus mucinosis
- Alopecia mucinosa

LABORATORY WORK-UP
- Skin biopsy for routine histology w/ mucin stains

MANAGEMENT
- Antimalarial agents
- Pulse dye laser

SPECIFIC THERAPY
- Hydroxychloroquine 200 mg PO BID for at least 2 months

CAVEATS AND PITFALLS
- Check for possible retinal toxicity of hydroxychloroquine if the drug is used for >6 months.

ROCKY MOUNTAIN SPOTTED FEVER

ALTERNATE DISEASE NAME
- Tick fever
- Spotted fever
- Tick typhus
- New World spotted fever
- Sao Paulo fever

HISTORY
- Fever, headache occurring within 1–2 weeks of tick bite
- Other presenting signs & symptoms include GI disturbances, malaise, myalgias, anorexia, irritability & photophobia

PHYSICAL EXAMINATION
- Skin & mucous membrane changes
- Rash beginning as confluent macular & papular eruption on wrists & ankles & spreading centripetally to trunk, proximal extremities & palms & soles
- Eruption becomes petechial after a few days
- Eye changes include conjunctival suffusion, periorbital edema & photophobia
- Cardiovascular changes include myocarditis, arrhythmias, occasional hypotension & congestive heart failure
- Pulmonary changes include pneumonitis & pulmonary edema in severe cases
- GI changes include anorexia, abdominal pain & tenderness, diarrhea, jaundice in severe cases, hepatomegaly & splenomegaly
- Musculoskeletal changes include myalgia, especially in legs, abdomen & back, diffuse arthralgias, edema on dorsum of hands & feet
- CNS changes include restlessness & irritability, altered mental status signs of meningoencephalitis, cranial neuropathies, paralysis, ataxia & meningismus

DIFFERENTIAL DIAGNOSIS
- Meningococcemia or other forms of bacterial sepsis
- Toxic shock syndrome
- Other rickettsial infections
- Lyme disease
- Drug hypersensitivity
- Infectious mononucleosis
- Babesiosis
- Ehrlichiosis
- Leptospirosis
- Malaria
- Dengue fever

- Rubeola
- Tularemia
- Allergic vasculitis
- Brill-Zinsser disease
- Atypical measles

LABORATORY WORK-UP
- Indirect fluorescent antibody test
- Skin biopsy w/ Giemsa staining, looking for organism

MANAGEMENT
- Systemic antibiotics

SPECIFIC THERAPY
- Doxycycline 100 mg PO BID for 7 days & for at least 48 hours after defervescence
- Chloramphenicol: adult dose, 500 mg IV divided into 4 doses per day for 7 days; pediatric dose, 50 mg/kg PO divided into 4 doses for 7 days & for at least 48 hours after defervescence

CAVEATS AND PITFALLS
- None

ROSACEA

ALTERNATE DISEASE NAME
- Acne rosacea

HISTORY
- Background of frequent facial flushing
- Worsened by any activity that produces flushing such as hot beverages, spicy foods, alcohol consumption & sunlight exposure

PHYSICAL EXAMINATION
- Erythema & telangiectasia over cheeks & forehead
- Inflammatory papules & pustules, predominantly over nose, forehead & cheeks
- Extrafacial involvement over neck & upper chest
- Prominent sebaccous glands w/ development of thickened & disfigured nose (rhinophyma)

- Ocular variant: conjunctival injection, chalazion & episcleritis
- Granulomatous variant (lupus miliaris disseminata faciei): inflammatory, erythematous or flesh-colored papules distributed symmetrically across upper face, particularly around eyes & nose

DIFFERENTIAL DIAGNOSIS
- Seborrheic dermatitis
- Acne vulgaris
- Perioral dermatitis
- Lupus erythematosus
- Polymorphous light eruption
- Tinea faciei
- Folliculitis
- Lupus vulgaris
- Carcinoid syndrome

LABORATORY WORK-UP
- None

MANAGEMENT
- Systemic antibiotics used as anti-inflammatory agents
- Topical anti-inflammatory agents
- Topical retinoids
- Systemic retinoids
- Pulsed dye laser or intense pulse light (IPL) ablation of telangiectasias
- Dermabrasion or laser abrasion for rhinophyma

SPECIFIC THERAPY
- Tetracycline 250–500 mg PO BID
- Minocycline 50–100 mg PO BID
- Doxycycline 100–200 mg PO QD
- Metronidazole 0.75% gel applied QD
- Azelaic acid 15–20% applied BID
- Tretinoin 0.025% cream applied QD
- Isotretinoin 10 mg PO QD for 4–6 months

CAVEATS AND PITFALLS
- Systemic antibiotics used as anti-inflammatory agents
- Systemic retinoids contraindicated in pregnant women

ROSEOLA

ALTERNATE DISEASE NAME
- Roseola infantum
- Exanthem subitum
- Sixth disease

HISTORY
- Most primary infections asymptomatic
- 9- to 12-month-old child in previously good health who has abrupt onset of high fever (40°C) lasting for 3 days, w/ non-specific complaints
- May develop febrile seizures

PHYSICAL EXAMINATION
- With rapid defervescence of fever, onset of pink morbilliform exanthem composed of either discrete, small pale pink papules or a blanchable exanthem, lasting 2 days
- Enanthem (Nagayama's spots) consisting of red papules on mucosa of soft palate & base of uvula

DIFFERENTIAL DIAGNOSIS
- Other viral exanthems, including mononucleosis, rubeola & rubella
- Scarlet fever
- Meningococcemia
- Medication reaction
- Dengue fever

LABORATORY WORK-UP
- None

MANAGEMENT
- Antipyretic therapy such as acetaminophen

SPECIFIC THERAPY
- See "Management"

CAVEATS AND PITFALLS
- Therapy w/ foscarnet, ganciclovir or cidofovir may be indicated in immunocompromised pts.

RUBELLA

ALTERNATE DISEASE NAME
- German measles
- Three-day measles

HISTORY
- Spread by nasal droplet infection
- Incubation period of 14–19 days, w/ onset of rash usually on the 15th day
- Disease contagious from a few days before to 5–7 days after appearance of exanthem
- Most contagious when rash is erupting
- May have no prodrome in children, w/ rash being first manifestation; in adults, fever, sore throat & rhinitis often appear before rash

PHYSICAL EXAMINATION
- Exanthem starts as discrete macules on face that spread to neck, trunk & extremities, w/ coalescence into plaques
- Exanthem lasts 1–3 days, first leaving the face, often followed by desquamation
- Nonspecific enanthem (Forscheimer's spots) of pinpoint red macules & petechiae over soft palate & uvula just before or with exanthem
- Generalized tender lymphadenopathy involving all nodes, but most prominent in suboccipital, postauricular & anterior & posterior cervical nodes
- Adults may have joint symptoms
- Congenital rubella syndrome in infants whose mothers contract the disease during first trimester
  - Purpura at birth
  - Low birth weight; small head size; lethargy; irritability; deafness; seizures
  - Developmental delay & mental retardation

DIFFERENTIAL DIAGNOSIS
- Rubeola
- Other viral exanthems

- Scarlet fever
- Kawasaki disease
- Drug eruption
- Juvenile rheumatoid arthritis

LABORATORY WORK-UP
- None

MANAGEMENT
- Isolation for 7 days after onset of eruption

SPECIFIC THERAPY
- None

CAVEATS AND PITFALLS
- None

RUBEOLA

ALTERNATE DISEASE NAME
- Measles
- Rubeola morbilli
- Rubeola measles

HISTORY
- Incubation period 7–14 days (average 10–11 days)
- Communicable from just before onset of prodromal symptoms until approximately 4 days following onset of exanthem
- Prodrome consists of fever, photophobia, cough, coryza & conjunctivitis

PHYSICAL EXAMINATION
- Enanthem (Koplik spots)
- Blue-white spots surrounded by red halo that appear on buccal mucosa opposite premolar teeth
- Precedes exanthem by 24–48 hours & lasts 2–4 days
- Exanthem
- Starts on fourth or fifth day following onset of symptoms as slightly elevated papules, which begin on face & behind ears & spread to trunk & extremities within 24–36 hours

- Initial color is dark red; slowly fades to purplish hue & then to yellow/brown lesions w/ fine scale over the following 5–10 days

DIFFERENTIAL DIAGNOSIS
- Other viral exanthems, such as rubella, enterovirus, echovirus & cytomegalovirus infection
- Kawasaki disease
- Drug eruption
- Primary HIV disease
- Brucellosis

LABORATORY WORK-UP
- None

MANAGEMENT
- No specific therapy

SPECIFIC THERAPY
- None

CAVEATS AND PITFALLS
- None

SARCOIDOSIS

ALTERNATE DISEASE NAME
- Boeck's sarcoid
- Angiolupoid sarcoid
- Besnier-Boeck-Schaumann disease

HISTORY
- Most commonly presents in winter early spring
- May have constitutional symptoms, such as fever, fatigue weight loss
- Skin involvement usually accompanies signs of systemic disease, but it may occur w/out other signs of disease

PHYSICAL EXAMINATION
- Skin
  - Asymptomatic, red-brown macules papules, commonly involving face, periorbital, nasolabial folds extensor surfaces of extremities

> Round to oval, red-brown to purple, infiltrated plaques, the center of which may be atrophic
> Nontender, firm, oval, flesh-colored or violaceous nodules on extremities or trunk (Darier-Roussy sarcoidosis)
> Infiltration of scars
- Pulmonary system: dyspnea; dry cough; chest tightness or pain
- Lymphatic system: palpable lymph nodes
- Ocular involvement: anterior uveitis, associated w/ fever parotid swelling (uveoparotid fever)
- Neurologic
  > CNS involvement may be fatal
  > Seventh cranial nerve palsy most frequent finding
- Miscellaneous findings include myocardial involvement, arthritis, proximal muscle weakness renal failure

DIFFERENTIAL DIAGNOSIS
- Tuberculosis
- Lymphoma
- Pseudolymphoma
- Granuloma annulare
- Granuloma faciei
- Foreign body granuloma
- Drug reaction
- Lichen planus
- Lupus erythematosus
- Leprosy
- Syphilis
- Psoriasis
- Tinea corporis
- Necrobiosis lipoidica

LABORATORY WORK-UP
- CBC, serum chemistries
- 24-hour urine calcium level
- Skin biopsy
- Chest radiograph
- Pulmonary function studies if there are symptoms suggestive of pulmonary insufficiency
- Bronchoalveolar lavage w/ a CD4/CD8 ratio

MANAGEMENT
- Topical corticosteroids
- Intralesional corticosteroids for localized lesions
- Antimalarials
- Methotrexate
- TNF-alpha inhibitors
- Systemic corticosteroids only for serious systemic involvement

SPECIFIC THERAPY
- Clobetasol 0.05% cream applied BID
- Triamcinolone 3 mg/mL intralesional
- Methotrexate 5–25 mg PO weekly
- Azathioprine 2–3 mg/kg PO QD
- Hydroxychloroquine 200 mg PO BID
- Prednisone 1 mg/kg PO QAM
- Etanercept 50 mg SQ BIW for 3 months

CAVEATS AND PITFALLS
- If prednisone is to be used for >21 days per course of therapy, obtain baseline chest radiograph, TB skin test bone mineral density determination.
- Check thiopurine methyltransferase levels before starting azathioprine therapy.
- Check for possible retinal toxicity of hydroxychloroquine if the drug is used for >6 months.

SCABIES

ALTERNATE DISEASE NAME
- Seven-year itch

HISTORY
- Intense pruritus, particularly at night; close contacts w/ similar findings
- Crusted variant occurs in immunocompromised & institutionalized pts.

PHYSICAL EXAMINATION
- Slightly elevated, pink-white, linear, curved, or s-shaped line (burrow), located in webbed spaces of fingers, flexor surfaces of

wrists, elbows, axillae, belt line, feet & scrotum in men & areolae in women
- Burrows on palms & soles in infants
- Vesicles appear as discrete lesions filled w/ serous rather than purulent fluid
- Red papules on penile shaft
- Nodular variant: pink, tan, brown or red nodules lasting for many weeks
- Crusted (Norwegian) variant: minimally pruritic, hyperkeratotic, crusted plaques over large areas; prominent nail dystrophy & scalp lesions

DIFFERENTIAL DIAGNOSIS
- Atopic dermatitis
- Animal scabies
- Insect bite reaction
- Pediculosis
- Delusions of parasitosis
- Dermatitis herpetiformis
- Pityriasis lichenoides
- Lichen planus
- Contact dermatitis
- Psoriasis
- Ecthyma
- Impetigo
- Xerotic eczema
- Transient acantholytic dermatosis
- Linear IgA bullous dermatosis
- Seborrheic dermatitis
- Erythroderma from other causes
- Langerhans cell histiocytosis
- Fiberglass dermatitis
- Dyshidrotic eczema
- Pityriasis rosea
- Metabolic pruritus

LABORATORY WORK-UP
- Microscopic examination of burrow contents, looking for organisms or excrement

MANAGEMENT
- Permethrin
- Ivermectin
- Prednisone for severe associated symptoms

SPECIFIC THERAPY
- Permethrin 5% cream applied from neck downward; repeat in 7 days
- Ivermectin 200 mcg/kg PO; repeat in 7 days
- Prednisone 1 mg/kg PO for 5–10 days

CAVEATS AND PITFALLS
- Treat asymptomatic household contacts.
- If more than one resident of group home or nursing home unit is affected, treat all residents & staff.

SCARLET FEVER

ALTERNATE DISEASE NAME
- Scarlatina

HISTORY
- Associated w/ streptococcal infection at another anatomic site, usually tonsils or pharynx
- Abrupt onset of fever, headache, vomiting, malaise, chills & sore throat, w/ rash appearing after 1–4 days

PHYSICAL EXAMINATION
- Mucous membranes bright red, w/ scattered petechiae & small, red papules on soft palate
- During first days of infection, white membrane coating on tongue through which edematous, red papillae protrude (white strawberry tongue); after white membrane sloughs, tongue is red w/ prominent papillae (red strawberry tongue)
- Exanthem consisting of fine red, punctate papules, appearing within 1–4 days following the onset of illness; first appearing on upper trunk & axillae & then becoming generalized, w/ accentuation in flexural areas
- Eruption may appear more intense at dependent sites & sites of pressure, such as buttocks

- Sandpaper feel to affected skin
- Transverse areas of hyperpigmentation w/ petechiae in axillary, antecubital & inguinal areas (Pastia lines)
- Flushed face w/ circumoral pallor; rash fading w/ fine desquamation after 4–5 days

DIFFERENTIAL DIAGNOSIS
- Viral exanthem, including rubella, rubeola, fifth disease
- Toxic shock syndrome
- Kawasaki syndrome
- Drug reaction
- Lupus erythematosus

LABORATORY WORK-UP
- Cultures of infected oropharynx or other infected sites

MANAGEMENT
- Systemic antibiotics

SPECIFIC THERAPY
- Penicillin VK 500 mg QID for 10 days
- Benzathine penicillin G 1.2 million units as single IM injection
- Penicillin allergy
  - ➤ Cephalexin 250–500 mg PO QID for 7 days
  - ➤ Erythromycin 250–500 mg PO QID for 10 days

CAVEATS AND PITFALLS
- None

SCURVY

ALTERNATE DISEASE NAME
- Vitamin C deficiency syndrome

HISTORY
- Occurs only after at least 3 months of severe or total vitamin C deficiency
- Variable arthralgia, anorexia & listlessness
- Poor wound healing

PHYSICAL EXAMINATION
- Perifollicular hyperkeratotic papules, surrounded by a hemorrhagic halo
- Hairs twisted like corkscrews & may be fragmented
- Submucosal gingival bleeding
- Subperiosteal hemorrhage causing painful bones of legs and elsewhere
- Conjunctival hemorrhage

DIFFERENTIAL DIAGNOSIS
- Vasculitis
- Physical abuse
- Coagulation abnormalities
- Deep vein thrombosis

LABORATORY WORK-UP
- None

MANAGEMENT
- Ascorbic acid supplementation

SPECIFIC THERAPY
- Ascorbic acid 800–1,000 mg/day PO for at least 1 week, then 400 mg/day until recovery complete

CAVEATS AND PITFALLS
- None

SEABATHER'S ERUPTION

ALTERNATE DISEASE NAME
- Sea lice

HISTORY
- Onset few hours after ocean bathing

PHYSICAL EXAMINATION
- Pruritic papules in a bathing suit distribution pattern
- Occurs in axilla & on chest in men w/ significant chest hair

DIFFERENTIAL DIAGNOSIS
- Urticaria

- Cercarial dermatitis
- Insect bite reaction
- Scabies
- Folliculitis
- Jellyfish sting

LABORATORY WORK-UP
- None

MANAGEMENT
- Topical corticosteroids
- Antihistamines for sedation

SPECIFIC THERAPY
- Fluocinonide 0.05% cream applied BID

CAVEATS AND PITFALLS
- Treatment of minimal benefit in this self-limited process.

SEBACEOUS HYPERPLASIA

ALTERNATE DISEASE NAME
- Sebaceous gland hyperplasia
- Senile sebaceous adenoma
- Senile sebaceous hyperplasia

HISTORY
- Insidious onset of asymptomatic lesions on face
- More common in fair-skinned people, w/ a history of excess sun exposure

PHYSICAL EXAMINATION
- Well-demarcated, yellow to flesh-colored, dell-shaped papules
- Most commonly located on forehead & cheeks

DIFFERENTIAL DIAGNOSIS
- Basal cell carcinoma
- Fibrous papule
- Milium
- Molluscum contagiosum
- Syringoma

- Trichoepithelioma
- Sebaceous carcinoma
- Melanocytic nevus
- Sebaceous adenoma
- Sebaceous epithelioma
- Xanthoma
- Xanthelasma
- Squamous cell carcinoma
- Sarcoidosis
- Colloid milium
- Granuloma annulare
- Lipoid proteinosis

LABORATORY WORK-UP
- Lesional biopsy only if diagnosis is in doubt

MANAGEMENT
- Destruction by dichloroacetic acid, light electrodesiccation or liquid nitrogen cryotherapy
- Laser ablation; shave removal
- Isotretinoin for multiple lesions

SPECIFIC THERAPY
- Isotretinoin 20 mg PO 2–7 days per week

CAVEATS AND PITFALLS
- Therapy for cosmetic purposes only.
- Systemic retinoids contraindicated in pregnant women.
- Advise that there is prompt recurrence when isotretinoin therapy is discontinued.

SEBORRHEIC DERMATITIS

ALTERNATE DISEASE NAME
- Seborrhea
- Dandruff
- Seborrheic eczema
- Seborrhea capitis
- Pityriasis sicca

- Pityriasis simplex capitis
- Pityriasis oleosa

HISTORY
- More common in those who shampoo less frequently & in those under excess stress
- Associated w/ Parkinson's disease & HIV disease

PHYSICAL EXAMINATION
- Scalp changes vary from mild, patchy scaling to widespread, thick, adherent crusts
- Central facial erythema, scale, most prominent in skin folds
- Eyelids w/ poorly defined, scaly, reddish-brown plaques
- Poorly defined, red-brown, scaly papules & plaques in intertriginous areas, over presternal area & over central back

DIFFERENTIAL DIAGNOSIS
- Tinea capitis
- Atopic dermatitis
- Lupus erythematosus
- Rosacea
- Psoriasis
- Intertrigo
- Contact dermatitis
- Candidiasis
- Diaper dermatitis
- Pityriasis rosea
- Pityriasis lichenoides chronica
- Darier disease
- Hailey-Hailey disease
- Grover's disease
- Pemphigus foliaceous
- Xerotic eczema
- Chronic granulomatous disease
- Infectious eczematoid dermatitis
- Letterer-Siwe disease
- Staphylococcal blepharitis
- Tinea amiantacea
- Vitamin B and/or zinc deficiency
- Glucagonoma syndrome

LABORATORY WORK-UP
- None

MANAGEMENT
- Antiseborrheic shampoo, used daily
- Topical corticosteroids
- Seborrheic blepharitis: scrub eyelids daily w/ baby shampoo diluted 1:1 w/ water

SPECIFIC THERAPY
- Hydrocortisone 1% cream applied BID to face
- Triamcinolone 0.1% cream applied BID to body
- Betamethasone 0.1% lotion applied after shampooing

CAVEATS AND PITFALLS
- Most common cause of treatment failure is inadequate shampooing.

SEBORRHEIC KERATOSIS

ALTERNATE DISEASE NAME
- Seborrheic wart
- Senile wart
- Basal cell papilloma

HISTORY
- Slow-growing, asymptomatic lesions present on most adults after age 35–40 years
- Dermatosis papulosa nigra variant more common in blacks
- Rare variant w/ explosive onset of multiple lesions associated w/ internal malignancy (sign of Leser-Trelat)

PHYSICAL EXAMINATION
- Noninflamed, single or multiple, sharply defined, flesh-colored, light brown, gray, blue or black, flat papules, w/ a velvety to finely verrucous surface
- Edges raised off skin surface, giving lesion a "stuck-on" appearance
- Dermatosis papulosa nigra variant: small, pedunculated, heavily pigmented papule, w/ minimal keratotic element, on face

- Stucco keratosis variant: superficial, gray to light brown, flat, keratotic papules on dorsa of feet, ankles, hands & forearms
- Melanoacanthoma variant: deeply pigmented keratotic plaque

DIFFERENTIAL DIAGNOSIS
- Melanocytic nevus
- Melanoma
- Acrochordon
- Wart
- Actinic keratosis
- Basal cell carcinoma
- Squamous cell carcinoma
- Psoriasis
- Pemphigus foliaceus

LABORATORY WORK-UP
- None

MANAGEMENT
- Destructive modalities, including electrodesiccation & curettage & liquid nitrogen cryotherapy
- Shave removal
- Surgical excision

SPECIFIC THERAPY
- See "Management"

CAVEATS AND PITFALLS
- Treatment for cosmetic reasons only, except for irritated lesions.

SERUM SICKNESS

ALTERNATE DISEASE NAME
- None

HISTORY
- Associated w/ administration of foreign protein antigen, such as horse serum
- Fever, headache, myalgia, arthralgia & GI complaints

PHYSICAL EXAMINATION
- Urticarial, morbilliform or scarlatiniform or palpable purpuric eruption
- Pruritus & erythema at injection site
- Lymphadenopathy & splenomegaly
- Neurologic complications include headache, optic neuritis, cranial nerve palsies, Guillain-Barré syndrome
- GI complaints include abdominal pain, nausea, vomiting, diarrhea
- Clinical recovery after 7–28 days

DIFFERENTIAL DIAGNOSIS
- Urticaria
- Cryoglobulinemia
- Hepatitis
- Infectious mononucleosis
- Hypersensitivity vasculitis
- Lupus erythematosus
- Henoch-Schönlein purpura
- Still disease

LABORATORY WORK-UP
- CBC, urinalysis, serum complement, cryoglobulins

MANAGEMENT
- Antihistamines
- Systemic corticosteroids

SPECIFIC THERAPY
- Prednisone 1 mg/kg PO QAM for 7–21 days

CAVEATS AND PITFALLS
- Use systemic corticosteroids only in pts w/ significant systemic signs & symptoms.

SMALL PLAQUE PARAPSORIASIS

ALTERNATE DISEASE NAME
- Benign parapsoriasis
- Digitate dermatitis

- Digitate dermatosis
- Chronic superficial dermatitis
- Guttate parapsoriasis
- Brocq's disease

HISTORY
- Insidious onset of asymptomatic or slightly pruritic lesions
- Eruption may remain for many months, but may remit spontaneously

PHYSICAL EXAMINATION
- Well-circumscribed, slightly scaly, light salmon-colored papules or plaques scattered over trunk & extremities
- Digitate pattern: palisading, elongated fingerlike plaques following a dermatomal pattern, most prominently on flank

DIFFERENTIAL DIAGNOSIS
- Psoriasis
- Dermatophytosis
- Mycosis fungoides
- Xerosis
- Nummular dermatitis
- Lupus erythematosus
- Lichen planus
- Pityriasis rosea
- Syphilis
- Seborrheic dermatitis

LABORATORY WORK-UP
- Lesional biopsy

MANAGEMENT
- Topical corticosteroids
- Phototherapy

SPECIFIC THERAPY
- Fluocinonide 0.05% cream applied BID

CAVEATS AND PITFALLS
- Topical corticosteroids of marginal benefit.

SOUTH AMERICAN BLASTOMYCOSIS

ALTERNATE DISEASE NAME
- Paracoccidioidomycosis
- Lutz mycosis
- Brazilian blastomycosis

HISTORY
- Latency period of weeks to decades after exposure
- Constitutional symptoms include low-grade fever, malaise & weight loss
- Mucous membrane symptoms include pain at ulceration sites, particularly w/ eating or drinking
- Laryngeal & pharyngeal lesions can cause dysphagia, hoarseness or stridor
- Respiratory symptoms include cough, mucus production, which may be blood-tinged, & dyspnea

PHYSICAL EXAMINATION
- Adult chronic form
  - Slowly progressive, painful ulcerating papules or plaques in oral, nasal, pharyngeal & laryngeal tissue
  - Gingival lesions produce loss of teeth
  - Conjunctivitis & ulcerative lesions of perianal area
  - Skin lesions most often arise from direct extension of mucous membrane lesions, occur commonly on face
  - May be papular, nodular, ulcerated, papillomatous or tuberous
  - Hematogenous spread may produce widely scattered lesions & subcutaneous abscesses
  - Extensive hypertrophic, painful lymphadenopathy, w/ visceral & subcutaneous nodes
  - Node suppuration causes sinus tracts or skin ulcers
  - Clinical picture in lungs may resemble that of tuberculosis, w/ chronic dyspnea, cough & sputum production
  - Other systemic problems include hepatosplenomegaly, adrenal insufficiency, meningitis, intestinal ulcerations & osteomyelitis
- Juvenile subacute form
  - Mucous membranes rarely involved

> Acneiform eruption or subcutaneous abscesses
> Prominent lymphadenopathy w/ suppuration
> Scrofuloderma as a result of lymph node suppuration
> Mesenteric adenopathy may cause bowel obstruction

DIFFERENTIAL DIAGNOSIS
- Tuberculosis
- Actinomycosis
- Coccidioidomycosis
- Leishmaniasis
- Sporotrichosis
- Syphilis
- Histoplasmosis
- North American blastomycosis
- Wegener granulomatosis
- Carcinoma
- Drug eruption
- Lymphoma
- Leukemia

LABORATORY WORK-UP
- Wet preparation of exudate looking for organism
- Fungal culture

MANAGEMENT
- Systemic antimycotic agents

SPECIFIC THERAPY
- Trimethoprim/sulfamethoxazole DS BID for 2–3 years
- Ketoconazole 200–400 mg PO QD for 6–12 months
- Itraconazole 100 mg PO QD for 6 months
- Amphotericin B 0.7–1 mg/kg IV daily for 4–8 weeks, followed by trimethoprim/sulfamethoxazole for 2–3 years

CAVEATS AND PITFALLS
- Amphotericin B used only in severe, recalcitrant cases.

SPIDER ANGIOMA

ALTERNATE DISEASE NAME
- Spider nevus

- Nevus araneus
- Vascular spider

HISTORY
- Most often presents as isolated finding in otherwise healthy person
- Sometimes associated w/ pregnancy, oral contraceptive use & chronic liver disease

PHYSICAL EXAMINATION
- Red macule or papule surrounded by several distinct radiating vessels, occurring most commonly on face, below eyes & over cheekbones
- Blanching w/ central pressure

DIFFERENTIAL DIAGNOSIS
- Telangiectatic mat
- Spider telangiectasia
- Insect bite
- Cherry angioma

LABORATORY WORK-UP
- None

MANAGEMENT
- Destructive modality

SPECIFIC THERAPY
- Electrodesiccation
- Laser ablation

CAVEATS AND PITFALLS
- Treatment for cosmetic reasons only.

SPOROTRICHOSIS

ALTERNATE DISEASE NAME
- Rose gardener's disease
- Schenck's disease
- Beurmann's disease
- Peat moss disease

HISTORY
■ History of prick injury at site of infection, within 3 weeks of onset of signs & symptoms

PHYSICAL EXAMINATION
■ Lymphocutaneous variant
➤ Subcutaneous nodule developing at site of inoculation w/ ulceration after central abscess formation
➤ Satellite lesions form along associated lymphatic chain w/ regional lymphadenopathy
■ Fixed cutaneous variant: scaly, acneform, verrucous or ulcerative nodule remaining localized to site of inoculation
■ Disseminated variant: multiple organ involvement causing pyelonephritis, orchitis, mastitis, arthritis, synovitis, meningitis, bone infection or (rarely) pulmonary disease

DIFFERENTIAL DIAGNOSIS
■ Bacterial pyoderma
■ Atypical mycobacterial infection
■ Nocardiosis
■ North American blastomycosis
■ South American blastomycosis
■ Leishmaniasis
■ Herpes zoster
■ Foreign body granuloma
■ Anthrax
■ Cutaneous tuberculosis
■ Tularemia

LABORATORY WORK-UP
■ Fungal culture

MANAGEMENT
■ Systemic antifungal therapy

SPECIFIC THERAPY
■ Lymphocutaneous variant
➤ Itraconazole 100 mg PO BID for 4–8 weeks
➤ Saturated solution of potassium iodide (SSKI) 300–500 mg PO 3 times daily for 4–8 weeks

- Disseminated variant
  - Amphotericin B 3 mg/kg per day IV until significant clinical response
  - Itraconazole 200 mg PO BID indefinitely

CAVEATS AND PITFALLS
- Slowly titrate dose of SSKI over 1–2 weeks to minimize chance of overdose, often heralded by sneezing, nasal congestion & conjunctival irritation.

SQUAMOUS CELL CARCINOMA

ALTERNATE DISEASE NAME
- Epidermoid carcinoma
- Prickle cell carcinoma

HISTORY
- Often directly related to chronic sun exposure, particularly in fair-skinned individuals
- May evolve from pre-existing actinic keratosis

PHYSICAL EXAMINATION
- Elevated, firm, pink to flesh-colored, keratotic papule or plaque w/ or w/out overlying cutaneous horn or ulceration
- Lip lesion
  - Most commonly on vermilion border of lower lip
  - Shiny, ulcerated papule or nodule

DIFFERENTIAL DIAGNOSIS
- Actinic keratosis
- Basal cell carcinoma
- Benign adnexal neoplasm
- Melanoma
- Merkel cell carcinoma
- Atypical fibroxanthoma
- Seborrheic keratosis
- Wart
- Pyogenic granuloma
- Proliferating trichilemmal cyst
- Granular cell tumor

- Halogenoderma
- Infectious granulomatous diseases such as tuberculosis, leishmaniasis, coccidioidomycosis, North American blastomycosis & tertiary syphilis

LABORATORY WORK-UP
- Lesional biopsy

MANAGEMENT
- Surgical excision
- Destruction by electrodesiccation & curettage or liquid nitrogen cryotherapy
- Superficial orthovoltage radiation therapy
- Mohs micrographic surgery or other form of microscopically controlled excision for large tumors, lesions in anatomically sensitive areas or recurrent tumors

SPECIFIC THERAPY
- See "Management"

CAVEATS AND PITFALLS
- Metastatic potential increased in lesions >2 cm, mucous membrane tumors, or those that arise in chronic ulcers or chronic radiation dermatitis

---

STAPHYLOCOCCAL SCALDED SKIN SYNDROME

ALTERNATE DISEASE NAME
- SSSS
- Scalded skin syndrome
- Pemphigus neonatorum

HISTORY
- Original focus of infection often purulent conjunctivitis, otitis media or nasopharyngeal infection
- Prodrome of fever, irritability & generalized, faint, orange-red, macular erythema w/ cutaneous tenderness & periorificial & flexural accentuation

PHYSICAL EXAMINATION
- Early positive Nikolsky sign

- Rash evolves into generalized, superficial blistering eruption within 24–48 hours, w/ tissue paper-like surface wrinkling, followed by large, flaccid bullae in axillae & groin & around body orifices
- Mucous membranes spared
- After epidermal sloughing, moist erythematous base present, which heals within 5–7 days

DIFFERENTIAL DIAGNOSIS
- Toxic shock syndrome
- Kawasaki disease
- Scarlet fever
- Erythema multiforme
- Child abuse

LABORATORY WORK-UP
- Bacterial culture of involved skin
- Skin biopsy if diagnosis is in doubt

MANAGEMENT
- Systemic antibiotics

SPECIFIC THERAPY
- Dicloxacillin: body weight <40 kg, 12.5 mg/kg per day PO divided into 4 doses; body weight >40 kg, 125 mg PO 4 times per day

CAVEATS AND PITFALLS
- Children are much less ill than they appear; this differentiates it from toxic epidermal necrolysis.

STASIS DERMATITIS

ALTERNATE DISEASE NAME
- Venous eczema

HISTORY
- Associated w/ chronic edema of lower extremities
- Occurs commonly in those w/ history of deep vein thrombophlebitis or venous insufficiency

PHYSICAL EXAMINATION
- Acute flares w/ exudative, weeping plaques

- Long-standing lesions w/ lichenification & hyperpigmentation
- Medial ankle most frequently & severely involved
- Skin induration may progress to lipodermatosclerosis & violaceous plaques & nodules on legs & dorsal feet (acroangiodermatitis)

DIFFERENTIAL DIAGNOSIS
- Contact dermatitis
- Cellulitis
- Kaposi's sarcoma
- Atopic dermatitis
- Xerotic eczema
- Necrobiosis lipoidica
- Nummular eczema
- Dermatophytosis
- Benign pigmented purpura
- Pretibial myxedema

LABORATORY WORK-UP
- None

MANAGEMENT
- Topical corticosteroids
- Compression therapy w/ Unna boot dressings, controlled gradient compression device or compression stockings
- Systemic corticosteroids only for severe acute flares

SPECIFIC THERAPY
- Triamcinolone 0.1% cream applied BID
- Prednisone 1 mg/kg PO QAM for 7–14 days

CAVEATS AND PITFALLS
- Poor response to therapy if chronic edema is not aggressively treated w/ leg elevation, support hose & weight loss.

STEVENS-JOHNSON SYNDROME

ALTERNATE DISEASE NAME
- Erythema multiforme major

HISTORY
- Associated w/ recent infections, particularly herpes simplex virus infections, & medication

- Fever, cough or sore throat may appear 1–3 days prior to muco-cutaneous lesions

PHYSICAL EXAMINATION
- Erythematous papules, vesicles, bullae & target-like papules, mainly on face, trunk & mucous membranes, including oral & genital mucosa
- May involve linings of respiratory & GI tract
- Conjunctivitis w/ photophobia; burning sensation in eyes
- Systemic manifestations include hepatitis, nephritis, GI bleeding, pneumonia myalgia & arthritis

DIFFERENTIAL DIAGNOSIS
- Pemphigus vulgaris
- Aphthous stomatitis
- Herpes simplex virus infection
- Erosive lichen planus
- Toxic epidermal necrolysis
- Varicella zoster infection
- Behçet's syndrome
- Reiter's syndrome
- Bullous pemphigoid
- Henoch-Schönlein purpura
- Urticaria
- Viral exanthem
- Kawasaki disease
- Figurate erythema
- Fixed drug eruption
- Lupus erythematosus

LABORATORY WORK-UP
- Lesional biopsy
- Bacterial & viral skin cultures, if infection is suspected

MANAGEMENT
- Systemic corticosteroids

SPECIFIC THERAPY
- Prednisone 1 mg/kg PO QAM for 7–14 days

CAVEATS AND PITFALLS
- Most cases are self-limited w/out need for systemic corticosteroids, which are of only moderate benefit.

STEWART-TREVES SYNDROME

ALTERNATE DISEASE NAME
- Lymphangiosarcoma of Stewart-Treves

HISTORY
- Occurs at site of chronic lymphedema in an extremity
- Most common preceding event is mastectomy 10–15 years prior to onset of tumor

PHYSICAL EXAMINATION
- Violaceous patch that evolves into plaque or nodule in area of chronic lymphedema
- Palpable subcutaneous mass or poorly healing eschar w/ recurrent bleeding & oozing
- Nodules may become polypoid & develop small satellite papules
- Overlying epidermis may ulcerate

DIFFERENTIAL DIAGNOSIS
- Angioendotheliomatosis
- Angiolymphoid hyperplasia w/ eosinophilia
- Kaposi's sarcoma
- Lymphangioma
- Melanoma
- Metastasis
- Hemangioendothelioma
- Hemangiopericytoma

LABORATORY WORK-UP
- Lesional biopsy

MANAGEMENT
- Radical amputation of limb
- Radiation therapy

SPECIFIC THERAPY
- See "Management"

CAVEATS AND PITFALLS
- High metastatic potential.

STREPTOCOCCAL TOXIC SHOCK-LIKE SYNDROME DISEASE

ALTERNATE DISEASE NAME
- Strep toxic shock-like syndrome
- Streptococcal toxic shock-like syndrome
- Streptococcal TSS
- Flesh-eating disease

HISTORY
- May arise following minor trauma or from hematogenous spread of streptococcal infection from throat to site of blunt trauma
- Localized pain in an extremity, which rapidly progresses over 48–72 hours
- Rapid deterioration of general health w/ fever, hypotension, cardiomyopathy, nausea, vomiting, diarrhea, rhabdomyolysis, myalgias, muscle tenderness & weakness, acute renal failure, adult respiratory distress syndrome
- Laboratory abnormalities include elevated serum glutamic oxaloacetic transaminase (SGOT) & serum bilirubin, thrombocytopenia, leukocytosis, disseminated intravascular coagulation, hypophosphatemia, hypocalcemia & electrolyte imbalance

PHYSICAL EXAMINATION
- Localized edema & erythema w/ extreme pain & tenderness early in the course
- May become bullous & hemorrhagic
- May progress to necrotizing fasciitis or myositis & gangrene

DIFFERENTIAL DIAGNOSIS
- Toxic shock syndrome
- Stevens-Johnson syndrome
- Kawasaki disease
- Toxic epidermal necrolysis
- Gas gangrene
- Meningococcemia
- Staphylococcal scalded skin syndrome
- Drug reaction

- Scarlet fever
- Rocky Mountain spotted fever
- Leptospirosis

LABORATORY WORK-UP
- Culture of wound exudate
- Serial blood cultures

MANAGEMENT
- Systemic antibiotics
- IVIg
- Surgical debridement of necrotic tissue

SPECIFIC THERAPY
- Nafcillin 2 g IV q4h in adults; 100–200 mg/kg per day divided into 4–6 doses in children
- Clindamycin 600–900 mg IV q8h in adults; 20–40 mg/kg per day IV divided into 3 or 4 doses in children
- Intravenous immunoglobulin (IVIg) 1–2 g/kg over 2–3 days

CAVEATS AND PITFALLS
- Early surgical intervention is critical to survival.

STRIAE

ALTERNATE DISEASE NAME
- Stretch marks
- Striae distensae
- Striae atrophicans
- Striae rubra
- Striae alba

HISTORY
- Occurs during adolescence, pregnancy, or after topical or systemic corticosteroid therapy
- Associated w/ Cushing's syndrome

PHYSICAL EXAMINATION
- Flattened, atrophic skin w/ pink hue; lesions enlarge in length & width & become violaceous

- Older lesions are white, depressed, irregularly shaped bands w/ their long axis parallel to skin tension lines
- In pregnancy, lesions occur over abdomen & breasts
- Adolescent striae appear on outer aspects of thighs & lumbosacral region in boys & thighs, buttocks & breasts in girls
- Flexures affected w/ topical corticosteroid use, especially if used under occlusion

DIFFERENTIAL DIAGNOSIS
- Cushing's syndrome
- Linear focal elastosis
- Marfan's syndrome
- External trauma

LABORATORY WORK-UP
- If Cushing's syndrome is suspected, obtain 24-hour urinary free cortisol level & overnight 1-mg dexamethasone suppression test

MANAGEMENT
- Pulse dye laser ablation
- Topical immune modulators

SPECIFIC THERAPY
- Tacrolimus 0.1% ointment applied BID for at least 3 months

CAVEATS AND PITFALLS
- No reliably effective therapy.

SUBCORNEAL PUSTULAR DERMATOSIS

ALTERNATE DISEASE NAME
- Sneddon-Wilkinson disease
- Subcorneal pustulosis of Sneddon & Wilkinson

HISTORY
- Chronic relapsing, pustular eruption
- Some association w/ paraproteinemia, multiple myeloma, pyoderma gangrenosum, inflammatory bowel disease, rheumatoid arthritis

PHYSICAL EXAMINATION

- Variably pruritic, superficial, flaccid pustules on normal or minimally red skin, typically involving axillae, groin, neck & submammary regions
- Purulent material accumulates in the lower half of the lesions, giving them a "bag of fluid" appearance
- Lesions are isolated or grouped & may coalesce to form annular, circinate or serpiginous plaques, often w/ postinflammatory hyperpigmentation

DIFFERENTIAL DIAGNOSIS

- Impetigo or other bacterial pyoderma
- Pustular psoriasis
- Folliculitis
- Pemphigus foliaceous
- Pemphigus vulgaris
- Dermatitis herpetiformis
- Acute generalized exanthematous pustulosis
- Dermatophytosis

LABORATORY WORK-UP

- Lesional biopsy

MANAGEMENT

- Sulfones
- Systemic retinoids
- Phototherapy
- Topical corticosteroids

SPECIFIC THERAPY

- Dapsone 100 mg PO QD; titrate as per response to therapy
- Acitretin 25–75 mg PO QD

CAVEATS AND PITFALLS

- Check CBC Q2–3 weeks for 10–12 weeks w/ dapsone to detect rare pancytopenia.
- Obtain baseline G6PD level before dapsone therapy.
- Systemic retinoids are contraindicated in pregnant women.

SUPERNUMERARY DIGIT

ALTERNATE DISEASE NAME
- Rudimentary polydactyly
- Digital duplication

HISTORY
- Lesion is present at birth

PHYSICAL EXAMINATION
- Smooth, flesh-colored papule at base of fifth digit

DIFFERENTIAL DIAGNOSIS
- Fibroma
- Neuroma
- Neurofibroma
- Pyogenic granuloma
- Wart

LABORATORY WORK-UP
- None

MANAGEMENT
- Surgical removal

SPECIFIC THERAPY
- See "Management"

CAVEATS AND PITFALLS
- Surgical excision for cosmetic reasons only.

SUPERNUMERARY NIPPLE

ALTERNATE DSEASE NAME
- Accessory nipple
- Polythelia

HISTORY
- Present from birth
- Enlarges at puberty

PHYSICAL EXAMINATION
- Small, pigmented or pearl-colored macule or papule or concave or umbilicated papule
- May be distributed bilaterally or unilaterally, symmetrically or asymmetrically
- Usually located along milk line

DIFFERENTIAL DIAGNOSIS
- Nevocellular nevus
- Lipoma
- Wart
- Acrochordon
- Lymphangioma
- Neurofibroma

LABORATORY WORK-UP
- None

MANAGEMENT
- Surgical excision

SPECIFIC THERAPY
- See "Management"

CAVEATS AND PITFALLS
- Surgical removal for cosmetic reasons only.

SYPHILIS

ALTERNATE DISEASE NAME
- Lues

HISTORY
- Sexually transmitted disease
- Primary disease appears within 3 weeks of contact w/ an infected person
- Secondary syphilis usually presents w/ a cutaneous eruption within 2–10 weeks after the primary chancre, often w/ mild constitutional symptoms & signs

PHYSICAL EXAMINATION
- Primary syphilis
  - Single ulcerated lesion w/ surrounding red areola
  - Ulcer edge & base have button-like consistency
  - Painless regional lymphadenopathy
  - Usually heals within 4–8 weeks
- Secondary syphilis
  - Bilaterally symmetrical, pale red to pink, discrete, round macules on trunk & proximal extremities
  - After several days or weeks, red, scaly papules appear, sometimes becoming necrotic
  - Distributed widely w/ frequent involvement of palms & soles
  - Small papular follicular syphilids involving hair follicles may result in patchy alopecia
  - Highly infectious papules develop at mucocutaneous junctions & in moist intertriginous skin & become hypertrophic & dull pink or gray (condyloma lata)
  - Superficial mucosal erosions on palate, pharynx, larynx, glans penis, vulva & in anal canal & rectum (mucous patches)
- Late syphilis
  - Usually solitary gummas present as indurated, nodular, papulosquamous or ulcerative lesions forming circles or arcs w/ peripheral hyperpigmentation
  - Cardiovascular findings include diastolic murmur w/ a tambour quality, secondary to aortic dilation w/ valvular insufficiency
  - Symptomatic neurosyphilis findings include meningovascular lesions; cranial nerve palsies & pupillary abnormalities, tabes dorsalis & feet ulcers from loss of pain sensation
- Congenital syphilis
  - Early manifestations include diffuse eruption, w/ sloughing of epithelium, particularly on palms, soles & skin around mouth & anus
  - Miscellaneous findings include hepatomegaly; splenomegaly; petechiae, anemia, lymphadenopathy, jaundice, pseudoparalysis, snuffles, depressed linear scars radiating from orifice of mouth (rhagades or Parrot lines)
  - Late manifestations include interstitial keratitis, cranial nerve deafness, corneal opacities & recurrent arthropathy

> Clinical manifestations of untreated congenital neurosyphilis include gummatous periostitis, saddle nose, dental abnormalities including centrally notched & widely spaced, peg-shaped, upper central incisors (Hutchinson teeth) & sixth-year molars w/ multiple poorly developed cusps (mulberry molars)

> Skeletal findings include frontal bossing & unilateral irregular enlargement of sternoclavicular portion of clavicle

DIFFERENTIAL DIAGNOSIS
- Tinea corporis
- Psoriasis
- Parapsoriasis
- Lichen planus
- Pityriasis rosea
- Chancroid
- Lymphogranuloma venereum
- Granuloma inguinale
- Herpes simplex virus infection
- Drug eruption
- Erythema multiforme
- Leprosy
- Amyloidosis
- Lupus erythematosus
- Sarcoidosis
- Traumatic balanitis

LABORATORY WORK-UP
- Darkfield exam of tissue fluid from primary lesion
- Serologic test for syphilis
- Lumbar puncture if late syphilis is suspected
- Bone radiographs in suspected congenital syphilis

MANAGEMENT
- Systemic antibiotics

SPECIFIC THERAPY
- Penicillin G benzathine 2.4 million units for primary or secondary disease
- Erythromycin 500 mg PO QID for 2–4 weeks for primary or secondary disease

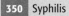

■ Tetracycline 500 mg PO QID for 14 days for primary or secondary disease

CAVEATS AND PITFALLS
■ Check for additional sexually transmitted diseases.

SYRINGOMA

ALTERNATE DISEASE NAME
■ None

HISTORY
■ Asymptomatic lesions that occur almost exclusively in adults

PHYSICAL EXAMINATION
■ Skin-colored or yellowish, small, dermal papules, often w/ a translucent or cystic appearance
■ Located most commonly on upper parts of cheeks & lower eyelids but also on axilla, chest, abdomen, penis & vulva

DIFFERENTIAL DIAGNOSIS
■ Trichoepithelioma
■ Basal cell carcinoma
■ Molluscum contagiosum
■ Milium
■ Flat wart
■ Xanthelasma
■ Granuloma annulare

LABORATORY WORK-UP
■ Lesional biopsy if diagnosis is in doubt

MANAGEMENT
■ Surgical removal
  ➤ Electrodesiccation & curettage
  ➤ Dichloroacetic acid application
  ➤ Dermabrasion
  ➤ TCA chemical peel

SPECIFIC THERAPY
■ See "Management"

CAVEATS AND PITFALLS

■ Surgical therapy for cosmetic reasons only

T-CELL LYMPHOMA, PERIPHERAL

ALTERNATE DISEASE NAME

■ Mycosis fungoides

HISTORY

■ Extended period of nonspecific signs & symptoms, pruritus being a common symptom

■ Many older pts have pre-existent adult-onset atopic dermatitis.

PHYSICAL EXAMINATION

■ Patch stage
  ➤ Flat, erythematous patches, sometimes becoming more infiltrative & evolving into palpable, scaly plaques w/ irregular borders
  ➤ Alopecia if scalp is involved

■ Tumor stage: red to violaceous, exophytic and/or ulcerated nodules, which may eventuate in generalized erythroderma

■ Pagetoid reticulosis (Woringer-Kolopp disease) variant: solitary, asymptomatic, slowly enlarging, well-defined, red, scaly plaque on extremities

■ Sézary variant: large number of circulating abnormal T cells w/ erythroderma & lymphadenopathy

DIFFERENTIAL DIAGNOSIS

■ Parapsoriasis en plaque
■ Lymphomatoid papulosis
■ Psoriasis
■ Lupus erythematosus
■ Lichen planus
■ Atopic dermatitis
■ Tinea corporis
■ Other causes of exfoliative erythroderma, including drug eruption, seborrheic dermatitis & pemphigus foliaceus

LABORATORY WORK-UP

■ Lesional biopsy for routine histology

■ Evaluate w/ immunopathologic techniques if routine exam is not diagnostic

MANAGEMENT
■ Topical/physical modalities
  ➤ Topical corticosteroids
  ➤ Topical chemotherapy
  ➤ Phototherapy
  ➤ Extracorporeal photopheresis
  ➤ Electron beam therapy

SPECIFIC THERAPY
■ Topical therapies
■ Mechlorethamine (nitrogen mustard)
  ➤ 10 mg dissolved in 60 mL water & applied daily
  ➤ 90 mg in absolute alcohol 10 & hydrophilic ointment QS 900 g
■ Carmustine (BCNU): 100 mg dissolved in 50 mL alcohol; 5 mL dissolved in 50 mL water for daily application
■ Systemic therapies
  ➤ Prednisone 1 mg/kg PO QAM
  ➤ Methotrexate 5–25 mg PO Q 1 week
  ➤ Isotretinoin 1–2 mg/kg PO QD
  ➤ Bexarotene 20–150 mcg PO per day
  ➤ Systemic chemotherapy

CAVEATS AND PITFALLS
■ No therapy affects the overall survival rate.
■ If prednisone is to be used for >21 days per course of therapy, obtain baseline chest radiograph, TB skin test & bone mineral density determination.

TELOGEN EFFLUVIUM

ALTERNATE DISEASE NAME
■ Telogen defluvium

HISTORY
■ Usually begins after a metabolic or physiologic stress 1–6 months before start of hair shedding

- Inciting stresses include febrile illness, major injury, change in diet, pregnancy & delivery & beginning a new medication
- Chronic form may be induced by chronic illness such as malignancy, particularly lymphoproliferative malignancy, & any chronic debilitating illness such as systemic lupus erythematosus, end-stage renal disease or liver disease, hormonal changes, diet changes & heavy metal intoxication

PHYSICAL EXAMINATION
- Acute form: relatively sudden onset of diffuse scalp hair loss
- Chronic form: hair shedding lasting >6 months

DIFFERENTIAL DIAGNOSIS
- Alopecia areata
- Androgenetic alopecia
- Anagen effluvium
- Trichotillomania
- Tinea capitis
- Traumatic hair breakage

LABORATORY WORK-UP
- None

MANAGEMENT
- Self-limited in most cases
- Topical minoxidil in recalcitrant cases

SPECIFIC THERAPY
- Minoxidil 5% solution 1 mL applied twice daily

CAVEATS AND PITFALLS
- Therapy not needed in most cases

TENNIS NAIL

ALTERNATE DISEASE NAME
- Sportsman's toe
- Tennis toe

HISTORY
- Occurs in those who participate in sports w/ quick starts & stops such as basketball, tennis, squash, racquetball

PHYSICAL EXAMINATION
- Pain & reddish-blue discoloration under affected nail plate
- Often affects either great toe or second toe, whichever is longer
- May appear w/ jogging & affect third, fourth or fifth toes, secondary to repeated pounding of foot on a firm running surface

DIFFERENTIAL DIAGNOSIS
- Melanoma
- Melanocytic nevus

LABORATORY WORK-UP
- None

MANAGEMENT
- Puncture of nail plate w/ a blunt pointed instrument, such as a heated paper clip, to express blood

SPECIFIC THERAPY
- See "Management"

CAVEATS AND PITFALLS
- None

TINEA CAPITIS

ALTERNATE DISEASE NAME
- Ringworm of the scalp

HISTORY
- Infection spread by fomites, including hats & combs
- Insidious onset of mildly pruritic scalp eruption w/ variable alopecia

PHYSICAL EXAMINATION
- Begins w/ red papules progressing to grayish, annular plaques, consisting of perifollicular papules, pustules w/ inflamed crusts, exudate, matted hairs & debris
- Black dot variant: infection w/ fracture of the hair, leaving dark stubs visible in follicular orifices

- Kerion variant
- Extreme inflammation associated w/ infection w/ boggy scalp & pustules
- May progress to patchy or diffuse hair loss w/ scarring alopecia
- Favus variant (tinea favosa): chronic infection, characterized by yellow, cup-shaped crusts (scutula), which surround infected hair follicles

DIFFERENTIAL DIAGNOSIS
- Psoriasis
- Seborrheic dermatitis
- Pediculosis
- Alopecia areata
- Traction alopecia
- Trichotillomania
- Folliculitis
- Secondary syphilis
- Bacterial pyoderma

LABORATORY WORK-UP
- Potassium hydroxide preparation of affected scalp site, including hair
- Fungal culture of hair

MANAGEMENT
- Systemic antifungal agents
- Systemic corticosteroids for kerion

SPECIFIC THERAPY
- Griseofulvin 20–30 mg/kg PO QD for 6–8 weeks
- Itraconazole 200 mg PO QD for 1–3 weeks
- Terbinafine 250 mg PO QD for 4–6 weeks
- Prednisone 1 mg/kg PO QAM for 7–21 days for kerion

CAVEATS AND PITFALLS
- Treatment failure may occur because of reinfection by fomites, such as shared hats & brushes.
- Do not use systemic antifungal therapy unless there is laboratory evidence of fungal infection (KOH prep or culture).

TINEA CORPORIS

ALTERNATE DISEASE NAME
- Ringworm

HISTORY
- May be contracted from contact w/ infected dogs & cats

PHYSICAL EXAMINATION
- Rapidly evolving, annular, erythematous scaly plaques
- Border may be crusted or vesicular
- Intense inflammatory response w/ zoophilic fungi (e.g., *M. canis*)
- Tinea manuum variant: diffuse erythema & scale of palm, extending onto dorsum of hand
- Tinea imbricata variant: scaly plaques arranged in concentric rings
- Majocchi granuloma variant
  - Granulomatous reaction secondary to fungal folliculitis, usually caused by *T. rubrum*
  - Plaques studded w/ follicular papules and/or pustules

DIFFERENTIAL DIAGNOSIS
- Tinea versicolor
- Psoriasis
- Granuloma annulare
- Seborrheic dermatitis
- Lupus erythematosus
- Bacterial pyoderma
- Candidiasis
- Erythema annulare centrifugum
- Sarcoidosis
- Contact dermatitis
- Superficial pemphigus
- Pityriasis rosea
- Syphilis
- Nummular dermatitis

LABORATORY WORK-UP
- Potassium hydroxide preparation of scale from affected site
- Fungal culture

MANAGEMENT
- Topical antifungal agents
- Systemic antifungal agents

SPECIFIC THERAPY
- Clotrimazole 1% cream applied BID for 3–4 weeks
- Terbinafine cream applied QD for 7 days
- Terbinafine 250 mg PO QD for 4–6 weeks
- Itraconazole 200 mg PO QD for 1–3 weeks
- Griseofulvin 20–30 mg/kg PO QD for 6–8 weeks

CAVEATS AND PITFALLS
- Do not use systemic antifungal therapy unless there is laboratory evidence of fungal infection (KOH prep or culture).

TINEA CRURIS

ALTERNATE DISEASE NAME
- Jock itch
- Crotch rot
- Tinea inguinalis
- Groin dermatophytosis
- Ringworm of the groin
- Gym itch

HISTORY
- Occurs almost exclusively in men
- Risk factors include visit to a tropical climate, wearing tight-fitting clothes for extended periods, sharing clothing w/ others, sports participation & obesity

PHYSICAL EXAMINATION
- Erythema w/ central clearing w/ hyperpigmentation & advancing scaly border in inguinal creases
- May extend distally onto medial thighs & proximally to lower abdomen & pubic area
- Scrotum is spared

DIFFERENTIAL DIAGNOSIS
- Candida intertrigo

- Erythrasma
- Psoriasis
- Seborrheic dermatitis
- Pediculosis
- Bacterial pyoderma
- Contact dermatitis
- Acanthosis nigricans
- Benign familial pemphigus
- Langerhans histiocytosis

LABORATORY WORK-UP
- Potassium hydroxide preparation of affected area
- Fungal culture

MANAGEMENT
- Topical antifungal agents

SPECIFIC THERAPY
- Clotrimazole 1% cream applied BID for 3–4 weeks
- Terbinafine cream applied QD for 7 days

CAVEATS AND PITFALLS
- None

TINEA PEDIS

ALTERNATE DISEASE NAME
- Ringworm of the feet
- Athlete's feet

HISTORY
- Chronic pruritic scaling of feet

PHYSICAL EXAMINATION
- Interdigital variant
  - Maceration, fissuring & scaling, most often between fourth & fifth toes, usually sparing dorsal aspect of foot
  - May extend to plantar surface of foot
- Moccasin (hyperkeratotic) variant
  - Symmetrical, asymptomatic or pruritic erythema w/ slight scaling
  - Dorsal foot spared, but may extend onto sides of foot

- Vesicular variant: painful, pruritic vesicles or bullae, most often on instep or anterior plantar surfaces
- Ulcerative variant
  - Rapidly spreading vesiculopustular lesions, often w/ secondary bacterial infection & occasional cellulitis
  - Lymphangitis, pyrexia, malaise

DIFFERENTIAL DIAGNOSIS
- Psoriasis
- Dyshidrotic eczema
- Atopic dermatitis
- Candidiasis
- Xerosis
- Bacterial pyoderma
- Contact dermatitis
- Erythema multiforme
- Syphilis
- Localized pemphigoid

LABORATORY WORK-UP
- Potassium hydroxide preparation of affected site
- Fungal culture

MANAGEMENT
- Topical antifungal agents

SPECIFIC THERAPY
- Clotrimazole 1% cream applied BID for 3–4 weeks
- Terbinafine cream applied QD for 7 days

CAVEATS AND PITFALLS
- Recurrence very common, even after successful treatment.

TINEA VERSICOLOR

ALTERNATE DISEASE NAME
- Pityriasis versicolor
- Chromophytosis

- Dermatomycosis furfuracea
- Tinea flava

HISTORY
- Risk factors include warm, moist climate & immunosuppression
- Tends to worsen in summer & improve in winter

PHYSICAL EXAMINATION
- Well-marginated, reticulated, finely scaly, oval to round, variably colored papules, coalescing into plaques
- Most commonly located over trunk, neck, chest, w/ occasional extension to abdomen & proximal extremities
- In immunosuppressed pts, lesions in flexural regions, face or isolated areas of extremities

DIFFERENTIAL DIAGNOSIS
- Tinea corporis
- Vitiligo
- Seborrheic dermatitis
- Parapsoriasis
- Psoriasis
- Confluent & reticulated papillomatosis of Gougerot & Carteaud
- Erythrasma
- Pityriasis alba

LABORATORY WORK-UP
- Potassium exam of scale from lesion

MANAGEMENT
- Systemic antifungal agents
- Topical antifungal agents

SPECIFIC THERAPY
- Ketoconazole 400 mg PO Q1 week for 2 weeks
- Clotrimazole 1% cream applied BID for 2–4 weeks
- Ciclopirox 1% gel applied BID for 2–4 weeks
- Terbinafine cream 1% cream applied BID for 1–2 weeks
- Selenium sulfide 2.5% lotion applied every other day for 2 weeks

CAVEATS AND PITFALLS
- Recurrences common, particularly in summer

TOXIC EPIDERMAL NECROLYSIS

ALTERNATE DISEASE NAME
- Lyell syndrome
- Acute disseminated epidermal necrosis
- Acute skin failure

HISTORY
- Usually related to drug ingestion, particularly nonsteroidal anti-inflammatory agents, anticonvulsants & certain antibiotics
- Few-day prodrome of malaise, fever, cough, sore throat, myalgia, rhinitis & anorexia

PHYSICAL EXAMINATION
- Skin eruption starts as morbilliform rash, which rapidly evolves
- Epidermal sloughing in sheets, leaving moist, denuded skin
- Positive Nikolsky sign
- Hemorrhagic crusting of lips & conjunctiva
- Pneumonia is a major complication

DIFFERENTIAL DIAGNOSIS
- Toxic shock syndrome
- Stevens-Johnson syndrome
- Kawasaki disease
- Staphylococcal scalded skin syndrome
- Exfoliative erythroderma
- Bullous pemphigoid
- Pemphigus vulgaris
- Paraneoplastic pemphigus
- Chemical or thermal burn

LABORATORY WORK-UP
- Skin biopsy if diagnosis is in doubt

MANAGEMENT
- Discontinue all suspect medications
- Intravenous immunoglobulin (IVIg)
- Plasmapheresis

SPECIFIC THERAPY
- Intravenous immunoglobulin (IVIg) 2 g/kg IV given over 3 days

CAVEATS AND PITFALLS
- Denuded skin needs same type of care given to those w/ extensive burns.

TOXIC SHOCK SYNDROME

ALTERNATE DISEASE NAME
- Staphylococcal toxic shock syndrome

HISTORY
- Acute onset of multiorgan illness w/ fever, hypotension, cardiomyopathy, nausea, vomiting, diarrhea, rhabdomyolysis, myalgias, muscle tenderness & weakness, azotemia, acute renal failure & adult respiratory distress syndrome

PHYSICAL EXAMINATION
- Diffuse macular erythroderma or scarlatiniform eruption
- Erythema & edema of palms & soles
- Hyperemia of conjunctiva & mucous membranes w/ strawberry tongue
- Delayed desquamation of palms & soles

DIFFERENTIAL DIAGNOSIS
- Streptococcal toxic shock-like syndrome
- Kawasaki disease
- Staphylococcal scalded skin syndrome
- Toxic epidermal necrolysis
- Drug reaction
- Scarlet fever
- Rocky Mountain spotted fever
- Leptospirosis

LABORATORY WORK-UP
- Vaginal cultures of postmenarchal women
- Bacterial cultures of recent surgical sites or traumatic wounds

MANAGEMENT
- Hospitalization of all suspect cases
- Systemic antibiotics

SPECIFIC THERAPY
- Nafcillin 1–2 g IV q4h in adults; 50–200 mg/kg per day divided into 4–6 doses in children
- Clindamycin 600–900 mg IV q8h in adults; 20–40 mg/kg per day IV divided into 3 or 4 doses in children

CAVEATS AND PITFALLS
- Recurrences fairly common, even after adequate therapy, especially in vaginal primary infections.

TRACTION ALOPECIA

ALTERNATE DISEASE NAME
- Traumatic alopecia marginalis
- Pressure alopecia
- Massage alopecia
- Ponytail band alopecia

HISTORY
- Occurs in those whose hairstyles cause pulling of the hair at the roots (corn-rowing, etc.)

PHYSICAL EXAMINATION
- Patchy areas of hair loss, w/ hair-pulling test resulting in detachment of >6 strands
- May have perifollicular erythema, scaling & pustules
- Marginal alopecia in temporal region or occipital area; w/ corn-rowing hairstyle, most affected area is immediately adjacent to braided region

DIFFERENTIAL DIAGNOSIS
- Alopecia areata
- Androgenetic alopecia
- Trichotillomania
- Tinea capitis
- Follicular degeneration syndrome
- Lupus erythematosus
- Telogen effluvium
- Anagen effluvium
- Syphilis

LABORATORY WORK-UP
- None

MANAGEMENT
- Discontinue hairstyling practices that exert traction on hair or otherwise traumatize hair.

SPECIFIC THERAPY
- See "Management"

CAVEATS AND PITFALLS
- Hair loss may be permanent.

TRANSIENT NEONATAL PUSTULAR MELANOSIS

ALTERNATE DISEASE NAME
- None

HISTORY
- Lesions present at birth, mostly in black children

PHYSICAL EXAMINATION
- Pustules & pigmented macules found mainly on chin, neck or forehead, behind ears or on trunk, palms & soles
- No systemic signs or symptoms

DIFFERENTIAL DIAGNOSIS
- Mongolian spot
- Acropustulosis of infancy
- Erythema toxicum neonatorum
- Neonatal acne
- Neonatal herpes simplex virus infection
- Miliaria
- Milia
- Impetigo
- Candidiasis

LABORATORY WORK-UP
- None

MANAGEMENT
- No therapy indicated in this self-limited process

SPECIFIC THERAPY
- None

CAVEATS AND PITFALLS
- None

TRICHILEMMOMA

ALTERNATE DISEASE NAME
- Tricholemmoma

HISTORY
- Asymptomatic, slow-growing papule and/or plaque on face, ear or upper extremity

PHYSICAL EXAMINATION
- Small, flesh-colored papules
- Lesions may enlarge into small plaques, particularly in nasolabial fold region, producing thick hyperkeratotic surface suggestive of wart

DIFFERENTIAL DIAGNOSIS
- Basal cell carcinoma
- Epidermoid cyst
- Wart
- Neurilemmoma
- Trichoepithelioma
- Trichofolliculoma
- Clear cell acanthoma

LABORATORY WORK-UP
- Lesional biopsy if diagnosis is in doubt

MANAGEMENT
- Shave removal
- Elliptical excision

SPECIFIC THERAPY
- See "Management"

CAVEATS AND PITFALLS
- None

TRICHOEPITHELIOMA

ALTERNATE DISEASE NAME
- Trichoblastoma
- Epithelioma adenoides cysticum
- Trichoepithelioma papulosum multiplex
- Sclerosing epithelial hamartoma
- Brooke tumor

HISTORY
- Single or multiple slow-growing papules, mostly on face
- Multiple lesions w/ familial variant

PHYSICAL EXAMINATION
- Round, skin-colored, firm papule or nodule, located mainly on nasolabial folds, nose, forehead, upper lip & scalp
- Occasional lesions located on neck & upper trunk
- Rare ulceration
- Solitary giant trichoepithelioma: large, polypoid tumor, usually in lower trunk or in gluteal area

DIFFERENTIAL DIAGNOSIS
- Basal cell epithelioma
- Colloid milium
- Cylindroma
- Angiofibroma
- Milium
- Pilar cyst
- Syringoma
- Trichilemmoma
- Microcystic adnexal carcinoma

LABORATORY WORK-UP
- Lesional biopsy

MANAGEMENT
- Solitary tumor: surgical excision or shave removal
- Multiple tumors: laser ablation or dermabrasion

SPECIFIC THERAPY
- See "Management"

CAVEATS AND PITFALLS
- None

TRICHOSTASIS SPINULOSA

ALTERNATE DISEASE NAME
- None

HISTORY
- Insidious onset in adult life

PHYSICAL EXAMINATION
- Dark, follicular plugs or papules, sometimes w/ protruding tufts or spines of fine hair
- Most commonly occurs on nose & upper trunk

DIFFERENTIAL DIAGNOSIS
- Comedonal acne
- Keratosis pilaris
- Lichen spinulosus
- Retained dirt

LABORATORY WORK-UP
- None

MANAGEMENT
- Depilatory wax or adhesive strips
- Drainage w/ comedo extractor

SPECIFIC THERAPY
- See "Management"

CAVEATS AND PITFALLS
- Usually poor therapeutic outcome.

TRICHOTILLOMANIA

ALTERNATE DISEASE NAME
- Chronic hair pulling
- Morbid hair pulling
- Compulsive hair pulling

HISTORY
- May be associated w/ other stigmata of obsessive-compulsive disorder or depression

PHYSICAL EXAMINATION
- Incomplete nonscarring alopecia, in relatively localized sites
- Geometric shapes of involved area, w/ broken hair
- Occurs most frequently in scalp, but sometimes involves eyebrows and/or eyelashes

DIFFERENTIAL DIAGNOSIS
- Alopecia areata
- Tinea capitis
- Androgenetic alopecia
- Syphilis
- Lupus erythematosus
- Monilethrix
- Traction alopecia
- Pili torti
- Temporal triangular alopecia

LABORATORY WORK-UP
- None

MANAGEMENT
- Selective serotonin reuptake inhibitors in patients unable to control impulse after understanding nature of disorder

SPECIFIC THERAPY
- Citalopram 20 mg PO QD
- Mirtazapine 15–30 mg PO QD

CAVEATS AND PITFALLS
- Psychological counseling may be needed, particularly in children.

TUBEROUS SCLEROSIS

ALTERNATE DISEASE NAME
- Tuberous sclerosis complex
- Epiloia
- Bourneville disease

HISTORY
- Familial clustering
- Some features are present from birth; many others are acquired over time

PHYSICAL EXAMINATION
- Skin lesions
  - Angiofibromas (adenoma sebaceum) often in nasolabial folds & on cheeks & chin
  - Periungual fibromas (Koenen tumors)
  - Connective tissue nevus (Shagreen patch), presenting as flesh-colored, soft plaque in lumbosacral area
  - Ash leaf-shaped macules on trunk or limb
  - Guttate leukoderma
  - Café-au-lait macules
  - Poliosis
- Neurologic changes
  - Tuberosclerotic nodules of glial proliferation in cerebral cortex, basal ganglia, ventricular walls
  - Epilepsy
  - Mental retardation
  - Other features include schizophrenia, autistic behavior & attention-deficit/hyperactivity disorder
- Miscellaneous findings include cardiac rhabdomyomas, aortic aneurysm, renal angiomyolipoma & renal cysts, pulmonary lymphangiomatosis w/ cyst formation, microhamartomatous polyps in bone cysts, pituitary adrenal dysfunction, thyroid

disorders, premature puberty, diffuse cutaneous reticulohisti-ocytosis & gigantism

DIFFERENTIAL DIAGNOSIS
- Acne
- Rosacea
- Connective tissue nevus
- Nevus anemicus
- Vitiligo
- Warts
- Trichoepithelioma
- Syringoma

LABORATORY WORK-UP
- CNS scans only if there are signs & symptoms suggestive of involvement

MANAGEMENT
- Destructive modalities for skin lesions, including laser ablation dermabrasion for cosmetic reasons only
- Genetic counseling

SPECIFIC THERAPY
- See "Management"

CAVEATS AND PITFALLS
- None

TWENTY NAIL DYSTROPHY

ALTERNATE DISEASE NAME
- Twenty nail dystrophy of childhood
- Trachyonychia

HISTORY
- Gradual onset in few nails, w/ more nails becoming involved over time
- More common in children, w/ tendency for improvement w/ increased age

PHYSICAL EXAMINATION
- Rough linear edges of nail plates
- Opalescent & frequently brittle nail plates that split at free margin

DIFFERENTIAL DIAGNOSIS
- Onychomycosis
- Lichen planus
- Psoriasis
- Onychophagia
- Traumatic nail dystrophy

LABORATORY WORK-UP
- None

MANAGEMENT
- No effective therapy

SPECIFIC THERAPY
- None

CAVEATS AND PITFALLS
- None

URTICARIA

ALTERNATE DISEASE NAME
- Hives

HISTORY
- Sudden onset of transient, pruritic lesions randomly distributed
- Associated w/ allergic reactions to many medications & foods
- Many cases of unknown cause

PHYSICAL EXAMINATION
- Edematous, pink or red papules or plaques (wheals) of variable size & shape, w/ surrounding erythema
- Angioedema variant: ill-defined, subcutaneous, edematous plaques, w/ associated pruritus, pain or burning sensation in lesions

- Dermatographism: urticarial wheal at site of light stroking or rubbing; may occur in pt w/ concomitant chronic idiopathic urticaria
- Pressure-induced urticaria: delayed response to pressure applied to skin
- Cold urticaria: wheal at site of cold application, which may also appear w/ rapid temperature change, w/out extremes of cold
- Solar urticaria: wheals after brief exposure to sunlight
- Cholinergic urticaria: small wheals triggered by heat, exercise or emotional stress
- Exercise-induced urticaria: wheals appearing after vigorous exercise
- Aquagenic urticaria: wheals appearing after exposure to water

DIFFERENTIAL DIAGNOSIS
- Urticarial vasculitis
- Erythema multiforme
- Insect bite reaction
- Mastocytosis
- Bullous pemphigoid
- Pruritic urticarial papules & plaques of pregnancy
- Melkersson-Rosenthal syndrome

LABORATORY WORK-UP
- Screening lab tests are of little value; order only those tests that will confirm clinical suspicion

MANAGEMENT
- Systemic antihistamines
- Recalcitrant disease
  - Systemic corticosteroids
  - Calcium channel blockers

SPECIFIC THERAPY
- Doxepin 10–25 mg PO HS
- Diphenhydramine 25–50 mg PO QID
- Prednisone 1 mg/kg PO QAM for no longer than 21 days
- Nifedipine 10 mg PO 2 or 3 times daily

CAVEATS AND PITFALLS
- Add calcium channel blockers only if antihistamines fail.

VARIEGATE PORPHYRIA

ALTERNATE DISEASE NAME
- Porphyria variegata
- South African porphyria
- Protocoproporphyria
- Mixed porphyria

HISTORY
- Chronic complaints of photosensitivity and/or ill-defined abdominal pain, or other constitutional symptoms
- Neuropsychiatric behavioral disorders
- Usual onset after puberty
- Familial clustering among certain families in South Africa

PHYSICAL EXAMINATION
- Skin manifestations
  - Photosensitivity
  - Skin fragility w/ noninflammatory vesicles & bullae, most commonly over dorsum of hands, w/ eventual scarring of sun-exposed skin
  - Hypertrichosis
  - Hyperpigmentation
- GI manifestations include abdominal pain & intermittent nausea & vomiting
- Neurologic manifestations include confusion, disorientation, agitation, psychotic behavior, seizures, coma & peripheral neuropathy

DIFFERENTIAL DIAGNOSIS
- Porphyria cutanea tarda
- Hereditary coproporphyria
- Erythropoietic protoporphyria
- Acute intermittent porphyria
- Pseudoporphyria
- Polymorphous light eruption
- Lupus erythematosus
- Epidermolysis bullosa
- Epidermolysis bullosa acquisita
- Drug-induced photosensitivity

LABORATORY WORK-UP
- 24-hour urine coproporphyrin & uroporphyrin taken during acute phase
- 72-hour stool collection for total fecal porphyrin

MANAGEMENT
- Acute attack management
- Strict avoidance of triggers, such as extreme carbohydrate-restricted dieting, certain medications, alcohol & smoking

SPECIFIC THERAPY
- Panhematin 3–5 mg/kg IV 1 or 2 times per day for 3–4 days

CAVEATS AND PITFALLS
- None

VARIOLA

ALTERNATE DISEASE NAME
- Smallpox

HISTORY
- 7- to 17-day incubation, followed by prodrome of fever, headache, pharyngitis, backache, nausea, vomiting & feeling of general illness

PHYSICAL EXAMINATION
- Oral mucous membrane enanthem
- Skin eruption starts w/ small, red macules on face & then spreads to extremities & trunk
- Lesions evolve into firm papules, then blister & develop into pustules, which form crusts & heal w/ pitted scars
- Lesions are typically in same stage of development
- Variola minor variant: constitutional symptoms, w/ fewer & smaller skin lesions

DIFFERENTIAL DIAGNOSIS
- Varicella

- Other viral exanthems, including coxsackievirus, parvovirus, infectious mononucleosis, rubella & rubeola
- Herpes simples virus infection
- Disseminated herpes zoster infection
- Impetigo
- Erythema multiforme
- Rickettsialpox
- Kawasaki disease
- Rat bite fever
- Leukemia
- Contact dermatitis

LABORATORY WORK-UP
- Swab of exudative material for viral identification

MANAGEMENT
- Immediately report any suspected case to state health officials & the CDC
- Strict respiratory & contact isolation for 17 days
- Vaccination in early incubation period for contacts

SPECIFIC THERAPY
- See "Management"

CAVEATS AND PITFALLS
- None

VENOUS LAKE

ALTERNATE DISEASE NAME
- Venous-lake angioma
- Senile hemangioma of lips
- Bean-Walsh angioma
- Venous varix

HISTORY
- Occur most commonly in adults >50 years w/ a history of chronic sun exposure

PHYSICAL EXAMINATION
- Well-demarcated, blue-purple, soft, compressible, smooth papules, typically over sun-exposed surfaces of face & neck, particularly on helix of ear, posterior pinna & vermilion border of lower lip

DIFFERENTIAL DIAGNOSIS
- Hemangioma
- Blue nevus
- Mucosal melanosis
- Melanoma
- Angiokeratoma circumscriptum
- Traumatic tattoo

LABORATORY WORK-UP
- None

MANAGEMENT
- Cryosurgery
- Electrosurgery
- Flashlamp pulsed-dye laser ablation
- Intense pulse light (IPL) ablation

SPECIFIC THERAPY
- See "Management"

CAVEATS AND PITFALLS
- Therapy for cosmetic reasons only.

VERRUCOUS CARCINOMA

ALTERNATE DISEASE NAME
- Carcinoma cuniculatum
- Epithelioma cuniculatum
- Ackerman tumor
- Ackerman's tumor
- Warty cancer

HISTORY
- Slow-growing verrucous tumor; may occur at site of chronic irritation & inflammation

PHYSICAL EXAMINATION
- Oral florid papillomatosis variant
  - Presents as white, translucent plaque on erythematosus base, located on buccal mucosa, alveolar ridge, upper & lower gingiva, floor of mouth, tongue, tonsil or vermilion border of lip
  - May develop in previous areas of leukoplakia, lichen planus, chronic lupus erythematosus, cheilitis or candidiasis
  - Lesions progress to white, cauliflower-like papillomas w/ a pebbly surface, sometimes extending & coalescing over large areas of the oral mucosa
  - May develop ulceration, fistulation, invasion locally into soft tissues & bone
- Anourologic type (Buschke-Loewenstein tumor)
  - Most commonly occurs on glans penis, mainly in uncircumcised men
  - May also appear in bladder & vaginal, cervical, perianal & pelvic organs
  - Presents as large, cauliflower-like lesion that may deeply infiltrate
- Palmoplantar variant (epithelioma cuniculatum)
  - Most commonly appears on skin overlying the first metatarsal head, but also may occur on toes, heel, medioplantar region & amputated stumps
  - Exophytic tumor w/ ulceration & sinuses draining foul-smelling discharge
  - Pain, bleeding & difficulty walking

DIFFERENTIAL DIAGNOSIS
- Wart
- Keratoacanthoma
- North American blastomycosis
- Leishmaniasis
- Leprosy
- Actinomycosis
- Tuberculosis
- Mycetoma
- Granular cell tumor

LABORATORY WORK-UP
- Lesional biopsy

MANAGEMENT
- Mohs micrographic surgery
- Destruction by electrodesiccation & curettage or liquid nitrogen cryotherapy
- Local radiation therapy

SPECIFIC THERAPY
- See "Management"

CAVEATS AND PITFALLS
- Recurrences common after incomplete excision.

WART

ALTERNATE DISEASE NAME
- Verruca

HISTORY
- Spread by both direct & indirect contact
- Autoinoculation may occur
- Very common in immunosuppressed pts

PHYSICAL EXAMINATION
- Common variant (verruca vulgaris): hard papules w/ a rough, irregular, scaly surface, most commonly seen on hands
- Palmoplantar warts
  - Begins as small, shiny papules & progresses to deep endophytic, sharply defined, round papules or plaques w/ keratotic surface, surrounded by a smooth collar of thickened horn
  - Plantar lesions usually found on weight-bearing areas, such as metatarsal head & heel
  - Hand lesions tend to be subungual or periungual
- Filiform variant: elongated, slender papules w/ filiform fronds, usually seen on face, around the lips, eyelids or nares
- Flat wart (plane wart, verruca plana) variant

> Flat or slightly elevated, flesh-colored, smooth or slightly hyperkeratotic papules, which may become grouped or confluent
> May occur in linear distribution as a result of scratching or trauma (Koebner phenomenon)
■ Mosaic variant: plaque of closely grouped warts, usually seen on palms & soles
■ Butcher's wart variant: verrucous lesions on hands, seen in people who handle raw meat
■ Condyloma acuminata (genital) variant
  > Pink to brown, exophytic, cauliflower-like papules or nodules on genitalia, perineum, crural folds and/or anus
  > Discrete, flesh-colored or hyperpigmented papules on shaft of penis
  > Lesions may extend into vagina, urethra, cervix, perirectal epithelium, anus & rectum

DIFFERENTIAL DIAGNOSIS
■ Seborrheic keratosis
■ Actinic keratosis
■ Squamous cell carcinoma
■ Acrochordon
■ Molluscum contagiosum
■ Prurigo nodularis
■ Callus
■ Arsenical keratosis
■ Lichen planus
■ Lichen nitidus
■ Acquired digital fibrokeratoma
■ Acne vulgaris

LABORATORY WORK-UP
■ None

MANAGEMENT
■ Keratolytic agent
■ Topical sensitizers
■ Topical or intralesional immunotherapy or chemotherapy
■ Hypnotherapy

■ Destructive modalities such as liquid nitrogen cryotherapy, electrodesiccation & curettage, laser vaporization or hyperthermia

SPECIFIC THERAPY
■ Salicylic acid 5–40% solution applied daily for weeks to months
■ Cantharidin applied once every 3–6 weeks
■ Squaric acid applied 1 or 2 times weekly after sensitization
■ Trichloroacetic acid 80% applied once every 4–6 weeks
■ Podofilox applied QD for 3 days per week for up to 4 weeks
■ Imiquimod applied TIW for 4–8 wk
■ Bleomycin 0.5–1 unit/mL intralesional injection

CAVEATS AND PITFALLS
■ There is no "treatment of choice" that is more effective than other therapies.

WEBER-CHRISTIAN DISEASE

ALTERNATE DISEASE NAME
■ Idiopathic lobular panniculitis
■ Relapsing febrile nodular nonsuppurative panniculitis
■ Nodular nonsuppurative panniculitis
■ Pfeifer-Weber-Christian syndrome

HISTORY
■ Crops of lesions that appear & resolve during a period of weeks to months
■ Systemic signs & symptoms include malaise, fever, nausea, vomiting, abdominal pain, weight loss, bone pain, myalgia & arthralgia

PHYSICAL EXAMINATION
■ Erythematous, edematous & tender symmetric, subcutaneous nodules, usually on lower extremities
■ Lesions resolve over a few weeks, leaving atrophic depressed scars
■ Occasional breakdown of nodules w/ discharge of oily liquid

DIFFERENTIAL DIAGNOSIS
■ Thrombophlebitis

- Vasculitis
- Sarcoidosis
- Erythema nodosum
- Erythema induratum
- Alpha1-antitrypsin deficiency panniculitis
- Polyarteritis nodosa
- Sweet syndrome
- Eosinophilic fasciitis
- Eosinophilic myalgia syndrome
- Leukemia and lymphoma
- Lipodermatosclerosis
- Pancreatic panniculitis
- Poststeroid panniculitis
- Scleroderma panniculitis
- Cytophagic histiocytic panniculitis

LABORATORY WORK-UP
- Lesional biopsy to include subcutaneous fat

MANAGEMENT
- Systemic corticosteroids
- Corticosteroid-sparing agents

SPECIFIC THERAPY
- Prednisone
- Corticosteroid-sparing agents
  - Hydroxychloroquine 200 mg PO BID
  - Azathioprine 2–3 mg/kg PO QD
  - Cyclophosphamide 100–200 mg PO QD
  - Mycophenolate mofetil 1,500–3,000 mg PO QD

CAVEATS AND PITFALLS
- If prednisone is to be used for >21 days per course of therapy, obtain baseline chest radiograph, TB skin test & bone mineral density determination.
- Check thiopurine methyltransferase levels before starting azathioprine therapy.
- Mycophenolate mofetil associated w/ fatigue & GI disturbances.

WEGENER GRANULOMATOSIS

ALTERNATE DISEASE NAME
- Wegener's granulomatosis
- Wegener's disease
- Systemic vasculitis
- Systemic necrotizing angiitis
- Necrotizing granulomatous inflammation of respiratory tract
- Necrotizing glomerulonephritis

HISTORY
- Presents w/ nonspecific constitutional symptoms & signs, often referable to upper & lower respiratory tract

PHYSICAL EXAMINATION
- Skin changes often over lower extremities
  - Palpable & nonpalpable purpura
  - Papules & subcutaneous nodules
  - Ulcerations resembling pyoderma gangrenosum
  - Vesicles, pustules & hemorrhagic bullae
  - Livedo reticularis
- Ocular findings: conjunctivitis, scleritis, proptosis
- Ear, nose & throat findings
  - Sinusitis & disease in nasal mucosa most common findings, w/ purulent or sanguinous nasal discharge
  - Otitis media
  - Deformation or destruction of pinnae or nose
- Oral findings
  - Mucosal ulcerations
  - Gingival hyperplasia w/ petechiae
- Renal findings: oliguria, hematuria, glomerulonephritis, w/ subsequent chronic renal insufficiency
- May also have cardiac & neurologic involvement

DIFFERENTIAL DIAGNOSIS
- Churg-Strauss disease
- Pyoderma gangrenosum
- Acute febrile neutrophilic dermatosis
- Polyarteritis nodosa

- Henoch-Schönlein purpura
- Cryoglobulinemic vasculitis
- Lethal midline granuloma
- Lymphomatoid granulomatosis

LABORATORY WORK-UP
- Skin biopsy
- Anti-neutrophilic cytoplasmic antibodies

MANAGEMENT
- Cyclophosphamide
- Systemic corticosteroids

SPECIFIC THERAPY
- Cyclophosphamide 100–200 mg PO QD
- Prednisone 0.5–2 mg/kg PO QAM

CAVEATS AND PITFALLS
- Check renal function & blood pressure regularly while on cyclophosphamide.
- If prednisone is to be used for >21 days per course of therapy, obtain baseline chest radiograph, TB skin test & bone mineral density determination.

XANTHOMA

ALTERNATE DISEASE NAME
- Xanthomatosis

HISTORY
- Familial clustering in hereditary hyperlipoproteinemias
- Prior history of myocardial infarction & other forms of atherosclerosis as well as pancreatitis in some of the syndromes
- Cutaneous manifestations may precede a diagnosis of hyperlipidemia

PHYSICAL EXAMINATION
- Xanthelasma palpebrarum variant
  - Asymptomatic, symmetric, soft, velvety, yellow, flat-topped, polygonal papules on & around eyelids, most commonly in upper eyelid near inner canthus
  - May or may not have associated lipid abnormality

- Tuberous xanthoma variant
  - Asymptomatic, firm, yellowish nodules usually developing in pressure areas, such as knees, elbows or buttocks
  - Associated w/ hypercholesterolemia & increased levels of LDL, w/ familial dysbetalipoproteinemia & familial hypercholesterolemia or w/ secondary hyperlipidemias (eg, nephrotic syndrome, hypothyroidism)
- Tendinous xanthoma variant
  - Slowly enlarging subcutaneous nodules around tendons or ligaments, often over extensor tendons of hands, feet & Achilles tendons
  - May appear after trauma
  - Associated w/ severe hypercholesterolemia & elevated LDL levels, particularly in type IIa form, or secondary hyperlipidemias, such as cholestasis
- Eruptive xanthoma variant
  - Sudden onset of crops of small, pruritic, red-yellow papules on an erythematous base, most commonly over buttocks, shoulders & extensor surfaces of extremities
  - May spontaneously resolve over several weeks
  - Associated w/ hypertriglyceridemia, particularly that associated w/ types I, IV & V (high concentrations of VLDL & chylomicrons) or w/ secondary hyperlipidemias, particularly in diabetes mellitus
- Plane xanthoma variant
  - Flat, yellowish papules, occurring at any site, occasionally covering large areas of face, neck, thorax & flexures
  - When palmar creases are involved, type III dysbetalipoproteinemia is the likely diagnosis
  - May also appear w/ secondary hyperlipidemias, especially in cholestasis, w/ monoclonal gammopathy & hyperlipidemia, particularly hypertriglyceridemia
- Xanthoma disseminatum variant
  - Appears in normolipemic adults as red-yellow papules & nodules w/ a predilection for flexures
  - May also appear on mucosa of upper part of aerodigestive tract
  - Usually resolves spontaneously

- Verruciform xanthoma variant
  - ➤ Normolipemic pts w/ predominantly oral cavity involvement
  - ➤ Solitary, papillomatous yellow nodule or papule

DIFFERENTIAL DIAGNOSIS
- Juvenile xanthogranuloma
- Amyloidosis
- Lipoid proteinosis
- Erythema elevatum diutinum
- Sarcoidosis
- Granuloma annulare
- Necrobiosis lipoidica
- Necrobiotic xanthogranuloma
- Calcinosis cutis
- Langerhans cell histiocytosis
- Rheumatoid nodules
- Gouty tophus
- Mastocytosis
- Lymphoma

LABORATORY WORK-UP
- Serum lipid profile; lipoprotein electrophoresis if screening tests are abnormal

MANAGEMENT
- Xanthelasma
  - ➤ Destructive modalities such as topical trichloroacetic acid, electrodesiccation or laser therapy
  - ➤ Surgical excision of isolated lesions
  - ➤ Control of underlying lipid defect or other illness causing lesions to arise

SPECIFIC THERAPY
- See "Management"

CAVEATS AND PITFALLS
- None

XERODERMA PIGMENTOSUM

ALTERNATE DISEASE NAME
- Kaposi's dermatosis
- Xeroderma of Hebra
- Angioma pigmentosum et atrophicum
- Atrophoderma pigmentosum
- Melanosis lenticularis progressiva

HISTORY
- May have early severe sunburns
- Some pts have history of consanguinity

PHYSICAL EXAMINATION
- Stage 1: diffuse erythema, scaling & freckle-like areas of increased pigmentation after age 6 months
- Stage 2: poikiloderma (skin atrophy, telangiectasias & mottled hyper- & hypopigmentation), producing an appearance similar to chronic radiation dermatitis
- Stage 3: appearance of numerous malignancies, including squamous cell carcinomas, basal cell carcinoma, malignant melanoma & fibrosarcoma
- Ocular findings: photophobia, conjunctivitis, eyelid solar lentigines, ectropion, symblepharon w/ ulceration, vascular pterygia, fibrovascular pannus of cornea & epitheliomas of lids
- Neurologic findings: EEG abnormalities, microcephaly, spasticity, hyporeflexia or areflexia, ataxia, chorea, motor neuron signs or segmental demyelination, sensorineural deafness, supranuclear ophthalmoplegia & mental retardation
- De Sanctis Cacchione syndrome: changes of xeroderma pigmentosum, neurologic abnormalities, hypogonadism, dwarfism

DIFFERENTIAL DIAGNOSIS
- Basal cell nevus syndrome
- Porphyria
- Bloom syndrome
- Cockayne syndrome
- Progeria

- Rothmund-Thompson syndrome
- Lupus erythematosus
- Polymorphous light eruption, including hydroa vacciniforme
- LEOPARD syndrome

LABORATORY WORK-UP
- None

MANAGEMENT
- Absolute protection from sun exposure from time of birth
- Surgical excision of skin malignancies
- Genetic counseling for families at risk

SPECIFIC THERAPY
- See "Management"

CAVEATS AND PITFALLS
- None

XEROSIS

ALTERNATE DISEASE NAME
- Dry skin
- Asteatosis

HISTORY
- Worsens w/ age
- Associated w/ atopic dermatitis in many pts
- Contributing factors include bathing in hot water, use of harsh soap, infrequent use of emollients, use of degreasing agents such as solvents or harsh cleansers & low environmental humidity w/ cold winds

PHYSICAL EXAMINATION
- Pruritus w/ or w/out associated skin signs
- Noninflammatory scaling, particularly over anterior legs & lateral arms
- May have eczematous changes w/ pattern of erythema craquelé, particularly on lower legs

DIFFERENTIAL DIAGNOSIS
- Ichthyosis vulgaris
- X-linked ichthyosis
- Atopic dermatitis
- Sarcoidosis
- Leprosy
- Cachexia
- Malnutrition
- Hypothyroidism
- Stasis dermatitis

LABORATORY WORK-UP
- None

MANAGEMENT
- Emollients applied at least BID
- Decreased bathing or showering
- Use of soap substitutes for cleansing
- Home humidifier, particularly in winter

SPECIFIC THERAPY
- See "Management"

CAVEATS AND PITFALLS
- None

X-LINKED ICHTHYOSIS

ALTERNATE DISEASE NAME
- Ichthyosis nigricans

HISTORY
- Onset at birth or in neonatal period
- Mother w/ asymptomatic corneal opacities

PHYSICAL EXAMINATION
- Adherent brown scaling in widespread distribution, producing dirty-appearing skin
- Scaling of scalp, preauricular skin & posterior neck
- Over time, scaling becomes more evident & assumes a dirty-yellow or brown color w/ dark, polygonal, firmly adherent scale

■ Flexures sometimes involved, but palms & soles usually spared

DIFFERENTIAL DIAGNOSIS
■ Ichthyosis vulgaris
■ Lamellar ichthyosis
■ Xerosis
■ Atopic dermatitis
■ Hygiene problem w/ resultant dirty skin

LABORATORY WORK-UP
■ None

MANAGEMENT
■ Emollients

SPECIFIC THERAPY
■ See "Management"

CAVEATS AND PITFALLS
■ Therapy is usually ineffective.

YAWS

ALTERNATE DISEASE NAME
■ Pian
■ Frambesia tropica
■ Bouba
■ Parangi
■ Paru

HISTORY
■ Usually a disease of children
■ Transmitted by direct contact w/ 90-day incubation period

PHYSICAL EXAMINATION
■ Primary stage
  ➤ Primary lesion (mother yaw) occurs at site of inoculation after a scratch, bite or abrasion, most commonly on legs, feet or buttocks

- ➤ Nontender, occasionally pruritic, red papule or nodule that ulcerates
- ➤ Satellite lesions may coalesce to form plaque
- ➤ Lymphadenopathy, fever & arthralgias
- ➤ Mother yaw resolves spontaneously in 2–9 months, leaving atrophic scar w/ central hypopigmentation
- ■ Secondary stage
  - ➤ Begins 6–16 weeks after primary stage w/ skin lesions (daughter yaws) resembling mother yaw but smaller
  - ➤ As lesions expand, onset of ulceration & exudation
  - ➤ Moist lesions in axillae, groin, mucous membranes
  - ➤ Papillomas on plantar surfaces
  - ➤ Macules or hyperkeratotic papules on palms & soles
  - ➤ Skeletal lesions include painful osteoperiostitis, fusiform soft tissue swelling of metatarsals & metacarpals
  - ➤ Relapses may occur after healing, up to 5 years following infection
- ■ Late stage
  - ➤ Begins after 5–15 years of latency w/ progressively enlarging, painless, subcutaneous nodules that ulcerate, w/ well-defined edges & indurated base w/ granulation tissue & yellowish slough
  - ➤ Keratoderma of palms & soles
  - ➤ Juxta-articular ulcerated gummatous nodules
  - ➤ Skeletal lesions include hypertrophic periostitis, gummatous periostitis, osteitis & osteomyelitis

DIFFERENTIAL DIAGNOSIS
- ■ Atopic dermatitis
- ■ Tuberculosis
- ■ Leishmaniasis
- ■ Leprosy
- ■ Psoriasis
- ■ Sarcoidosis
- ■ Scabies
- ■ Tungiasis
- ■ Warts
- ■ Syphilis
- ■ Keratoderma from other causes

- Insect bite reaction
- Nutritional deficiency

LABORATORY WORK-UP
- Dark-field microscopy of tissue fluid

MANAGEMENT
- Systemic antibiotics

SPECIFIC THERAPY
- Penicillin G benzathine 2.4 million units IM as single injection
- Erythromycin 500 mg PO QID for 14 days
- Doxycycline 100 mg PO BID for 15 days

CAVEATS AND PITFALLS
- None

ZOON BALANITIS

ALTERNATE DISEASE NAME
- Zoon's balanitis
- Plasma cell balanitis of Zoon
- Zoon's disease
- Zoon's plasma cell balanitis
- Balanitis circumscripta plasmacellularis
- Plasma cell balanitis
- Plasma cell mucositis

HISTORY
- Occurs almost exclusively in uncircumcised men

PHYSICAL EXAMINATION
- Solitary, shiny, red-orange to violaceous plaque of glans or prepuce

DIFFERENTIAL DIAGNOSIS
- Candidiasis
- Fixed drug reaction
- Lichen sclerosus
- Lichen planus
- Erythroplasia of Queyrat

- Syphilis
- Psoriasis

LABORATORY WORK-UP
- Lesional biopsy if diagnosis is in doubt

MANAGEMENT
- Circumcision

SPECIFIC THERAPY
- See "Management"

CAVEATS AND PITFALLS
- None

PART TWO

Therapy

ACITRETIN

TRADE NAMES
- No

GENERIC AVAILABLE
- No

DOSAGE FORM
- 10-mg, 25-mg capsule

SIDE EFFECTS, COMMON OR MILD
- Dermatologic: cheilitis, sticky skin, alopecia, xerosis, desquamation of hands & feet, pruritus, paronychia
- Eye: xerophthalmia
- Musculoskeletal: myalgias, arthralgias

SIDE EFFECTS, SERIOUS
- Reproductive: birth defects
- Musculoskeletal: spinal hyperostosis
- GI: pancreatitis, hepatotoxicity
- Neurologic: pseudotumor cerebri

DRUG INTERACTIONS
- Norethindrone
- Methotrexate

PRECAUTIONS
- Contraindicated in pregnancy.
- Use caution in pts w/ renal or hepatic dysfunction.
- Children may be more sensitive to bone effects, which may prevent normal bone growth during puberty.
- Advise about possible hyperlipidemia, especially w/ abnormal baseline level.

ACYCLOVIR

TRADE NAMES
- Zovirax

GENERIC AVAILABLE
- Yes

DOSAGE FORM
- 200-mg, 400-mg, 800-mg capsule
- 200 mg/mL oral suspension powder for IV solution

SIDE EFFECTS, COMMON OR MILD
- GI: nausea, vomiting
- Neurologic: headache

SIDE EFFECTS, SERIOUS
- Bone marrow suppression
- Neurologic: seizures, encephalopathy, coma
- GI: hepatitis

DRUG INTERACTIONS
- Aminoglycoside antibiotics
- Carboplatin
- Cidofovir
- Cisplatin
- Glyburide
- Metformin
- Mycophenolate mofetil
- Probenecid
- Nephrotoxic agents

PRECAUTIONS
- Use caution in elderly pts or those w/ renal insufficiency.

ADAPALENE

TRADE NAMES
- Differin

GENERIC AVAILABLE
- No

DOSAGE FORM
- 0.1% gel
- 0.1% solution
- 0.1% cream

SIDE EFFECTS, COMMON OR MILD
- Dermatologic: burning sensation, pruritus, erythema & scaling

SIDE EFFECTS, SERIOUS
- None

DRUG INTERACTIONS
- None

PRECAUTIONS
- Use caution when applying to eczematous skin.

AMITRIPTYLINE

TRADE NAMES
- Elavil

GENERIC AVAILABLE
- Yes

DOSAGE FORM
- 10-mg, 25-mg, 50-mg, 75-mg, 100-mg, 150-mg tablet

SIDE EFFECTS, COMMON OR MILD
- Dermatologic: dry mouth
- GI: increased appetite, constipation
- GU: urinary retention
- Cardiovascular: tachycardia
- Neurologic: confusion, dizziness

SIDE EFFECTS, SERIOUS
- Neurologic: seizures, cerebrovascular accident
- Bone marrow suppression

DRUG INTERACTIONS
- Acetaminophen/opiate combination drugs
- Alpha-2 agonists
- Amphetamines
- Antiarrhythmics
- Anticholinergics
- Other antidepressants
- Sedating antihistamines

PRECAUTIONS
- Avoid using immediately after myocardial infarction.
- Do not use within 14 days of MAO inhibitor use.

ANTIHISTAMINES, FIRST GENERATION

TRADE NAMES
(Generic names in parentheses)
- Benadryl, Dermarest, Sominex (diphenhydramine)
- Pyribenzamine (tripelennamine)
- Periactin (cyproheptadine)
- Phenergan (promethazine)
- Chlor-Trimeton, Comtrex (chlorpheniramine)
- Polaramine (dexchlorpheniramine)
- Atarax, Vistaril (hydroxyzine)
- Dimetane (brompheniramine)
- Sinequan (doxepin)

GENERIC AVAILABLE
- Yes

DOSAGE FORM
- Tablet
- Elixir
- Capsule
- Syrup

SIDE EFFECTS, COMMON OR MILD
- Dermatologic: dry mouth
- GI: diarrhea
- Neurologic: ataxia, dizziness, headache, agitation

SIDE EFFECTS, SERIOUS
- Neurologic: dyskinesia, seizures
- Respiratory: wheezing

DRUG INTERACTIONS
- Anticholinergics
- Antidepressants
- Antipsychotic agents
- Barbiturates

- Opiates
- Sedative-hypnotic agents

PRECAUTIONS
- Use caution in asthmatics.
- Excess sedation may impair performance of daily tasks.
- Paradoxical agitation may occur in small children.

ANTIHISTAMINES, SECOND GENERATION

TRADE NAMES
(Generic in parentheses)
- Allegra (fexofenadine)
- Claritin (loratadine)
- Clarinex (desloratadine)
- Zyrtec (cetirizine)

GENERIC AVAILABLE
- Yes

DOSAGE FORM
- Tablet
- Capsule
- Syrup

SIDE EFFECTS, COMMON OR MILD
- Dermatologic: dry mouth
- GI: nausea, diarrhea
- Neurologic: somnolence, fatigue, dizziness, agitation, headache

SIDE EFFECTS, SERIOUS
- Respiratory: hypersensitivity reaction, bronchospasm

DRUG INTERACTIONS
- Anticholinergics
- Antidepressants
- Antipsychotics
- Barbiturates
- Opiates
- Sedative-hypnotics

PRECAUTIONS
- Occasional sedation, particularly w/ fexofenadine
- Not usually helpful as antipruritic agent

AURANOFIN

TRADE NAMES
- Ridaura

GENERIC AVAILABLE
- No

DOSAGE FORM
- 3-mg tablet

SIDE EFFECTS, COMMON OR MILD
- Dermatologic: skin eruption, which may look like pityriasis rosea or lichen planus; stomatitis; pruritus; glossitis
- GI: diarrhea, abdominal pain
- Neurologic: change in taste sensation
- Eye: keratitis

SIDE EFFECTS, SERIOUS
- Renal: renal failure, nephrotic syndrome
- Pulmonary: pneumonitis
- Bone marrow: agranulocytosis
- Neurologic: seizures

DRUG INTERACTIONS
- Atovaquone/proguanil

PRECAUTIONS
- Dosage adjustments may be needed because of irregular GI absorption.
- Pt may develop anemia, leukopenia and/or proteinuria.

AZATHIOPRINE

TRADE NAMES
- Imuran

GENERIC AVAILABLE
- Yes

DOSAGE FORM
- 50-mg tablet

SIDE EFFECTS, COMMON OR MILD
- Dermatologic: alopecia, skin eruption
- GI: nausea & vomiting, diarrhea, dyspepsia

SIDE EFFECTS, SERIOUS
- Dermatologic: hypersensitivity reaction
- GI: hepatitis, pancreatitis
- Neoplastic: increased risk of neoplasm, particularly lymphoma

DRUG INTERACTIONS
- ACE inhibitors
- Allopurinol
- Cytotoxic chemotherapeutic agents
- Interferon
- Mycophenolate mofetil
- Warfarin
- Zidovudine

PRECAUTIONS
- Pt may develop asymptomatic liver enzyme abnormality.

AZELAIC ACID

TRADE NAMES
- Azelex
- Finacea

GENERIC AVAILABLE
- No

DOSAGE FORM
- 15% gel
- 20% cream

SIDE EFFECTS, COMMON OR MILD
- Dermatologic: pruritus; burning sensation shortly after application, dryness

SIDE EFFECTS, SERIOUS
- None

DRUG INTERACTIONS
- None

PRECAUTIONS
- None

AZOLE ANTIFUNGAL AGENTS

TRADE NAMES
(Generic name in parentheses)
- Exelderm (sulconazole)
- Ertacso (sertaconazole)
- Lotrimin, Mycelex (clotrimazole)
- Micatin (miconazole)
- Nizoral (ketoconazole)
- Oxistat (oxiconazole)
- Spectazole (econazole)

GENERIC AVAILABLE
- Yes

DOSAGE FORM
- Cream
- Solution
- Lotion
- Powder

SIDE EFFECTS, COMMON OR MILD
- Dermatologic: skin eruption, pruritus

SIDE EFFECTS, SERIOUS
- None

DRUG INTERACTIONS
- None

PRECAUTIONS
- None

BENZOYL PEROXIDE

TRADE NAMES
- Benoxyl, Benzac AC, Benza-Gel, Brevoxyl, Desquam-E, PanOxyl, Persa-Gel, Triaz
- Combination benzoyl peroxide products: Benzamycin, Benza-Clin, Duac

GENERIC AVAILABLE
- Yes

DOSAGE FORM
- 2.5%, 4%, 5%, 8%, 10% cream, gel, lotion, wash

SIDE EFFECTS, COMMON OR MILD
- Dermatologic: dryness, erythema & peeling, contact dermatitis

SIDE EFFECTS, SERIOUS
- None

DRUG INTERACTIONS
- Isotretinoin

PRECAUTIONS
- May bleach clothing.

CALCIPOTRIENE

TRADE NAMES
- Dovonex

GENERIC AVAILABLE
- No

DOSAGE FORM
- 0.005% cream
- 0.005% ointment
- 0.005% solution

SIDE EFFECTS, COMMON OR MILD
- Dermatologic: erythema, pruritus, irritant contact dermatitis

SIDE EFFECTS, SERIOUS
- None

DRUG INTERACTIONS
- None

PRECAUTIONS
- None

CAPSAICIN

TRADE NAMES
- Zostrix
- Zostrix HP

GENERIC AVAILABLE
- Yes

DOSAGE FORM
- 0.025% cream, gel, lotion, roll-on
- 0.075% cream, gel, lotion, roll-on

SIDE EFFECTS, COMMON OR MILD
- Dermatologic: burning sensation, erythema

SIDE EFFECTS, SERIOUS
- None

DRUG INTERACTIONS
- None

PRECAUTIONS
- Prolonged & severe burning sensation if applied to mucous membranes, such as the lip.

CEPHALEXIN

TRADE NAMES
- Keflex
- Keftab
- Bioccf

GENERIC AVAILABLE
- Yes

DOSAGE FORM
- 250-mg, 500-mg tablet
- 125 mg per 5 mL, 250 mg per 5 mL suspension

SIDE EFFECTS, COMMON OR MILD
- Dermatologic: skin eruption
- GI: nausea, vomiting, diarrhea
- Neurologic: headache, dizziness

SIDE EFFECTS, SERIOUS
- Immunologic: anaphylaxis
- GI: pseudomembranous colitis
- Bone marrow: thrombocytopenia, neutropenia

DRUG INTERACTIONS
- Aminoglycoside antibiotics
- Oral contraceptives
- Probenecid

PRECAUTIONS
- Pt may develop asymptomatic eosinophilia or elevated liver enzymes.
- 10–15% cross-sensitivity w/ penicillin.

CLINDAMYCIN, ORAL

TRADE NAMES
- Cleocin

GENERIC AVAILABLE
- Yes

DOSAGE FORM
- 75-mg, 150-mg tablet
- Intramuscular preparation
- Solution for IV injection

SIDE EFFECTS, COMMON OR MILD
- Dermatologic: skin eruption, pruritus
- GI: nausea, vomiting, diarrhea, abdominal pain, jaundice

SIDE EFFECTS, SERIOUS
- Dermatologic: anaphylaxis, Stevens-Johnson syndrome
- GI: pseudomembranous colitis, esophagitis
- Bone marrow: thrombocytopenia, granulocytopenia

DRUG INTERACTIONS
- Oral contraceptives
- Neuromuscular blockers

PRECAUTIONS
- None

CLINDAMYCIN, TOPICAL

TRADE NAMES
- Cleocin-T
- Duac (clindamycin & benzoyl peroxide)
- BenzaClin (clindamycin & benzoyl peroxide)
- Clindets

GENERIC AVAILABLE
- Yes

DOSAGE FORM
- 1% gel
- 1% solution
- 1% lotion

SIDE EFFECTS, COMMON OR MILD
- Dermatologic: burning sensation, dryness, scaling, pruritus, erythema

SIDE EFFECTS, SERIOUS
- None

DRUG INTERACTIONS
- Erythromycin, topical

PRECAUTIONS
- Rapid bacterial resistance if used w/out benzoyl peroxide

COLCHICINE

TRADE NAMES
- None

GENERIC AVAILABLE
- Yes

DOSAGE FORM
- 0.6-mg tablet

SIDE EFFECTS, COMMON OR MILD
- Dermatologic: skin eruption, alopecia
- GI: diarrhea, nausea, vomiting, abdominal pain
- Hematologic: anemia, thrombophlebitis

SIDE EFFECTS, SERIOUS
- Dermatologic: cellulitis
- Hematologic: agranulocytosis, aplastic anemia, neutropenia
- Neurologic: myoneuropathy

DRUG INTERACTIONS
- Cyclosporine

PRECAUTIONS
- Diarrhea is often first sign of toxicity.

CORTICOSTEROIDS, TOPICAL, HIGH POTENCY

TRADE NAMES
(Generic in parentheses)
- Cyclocort (amcinonide)
- Fluex, Licon, Lidex (fluocinonide)
- Topicort (desoximetasone)
- Diprosone (betamethasone dipropionate)
- Halog (halcinonide)

GENERIC AVAILABLE
- Yes

DOSAGE FORM
- Cream
- Ointment
- Lotion
- Gel

SIDE EFFECTS, COMMON OR MILD
- Dermatologic: skin atrophy, steroid addiction (rebound flare after discontinuing the medication), delayed wound healing, hypopigmentation, acneform eruption, striae

SIDE EFFECTS, SERIOUS
- Adrenal suppression

DRUG INTERACTIONS
- None

PRECAUTIONS
- Limit use on face to 14 days.
- Limit use in intertriginous areas to 1 week.

CORTICOSTEROIDS, TOPICAL, LOW POTENCY

TRADE NAMES
(Generic in parentheses)
- Hytone, Cortef, Cortaid, Texacort (hydrocortisone)
- Aclovate (alclometasone)
- Tridesilon, DesOwen (desonide)

GENERIC AVAILABLE
- Yes

DOSAGE FORM
- Cream
- Ointment
- Lotion
- Gel

SIDE EFFECTS, COMMON OR MILD
- Dermatologic: skin atrophy, steroid addiction (rebound flare after discontinuing the medication), delayed wound healing, hypopigmentation, acneform eruption, striae

SIDE EFFECTS, SERIOUS
- Adrenal insufficiency (very rare)

DRUG INTERACTIONS
- None

PRECAUTIONS
- Tachyphylaxis if used more than twice daily for prolonged periods
- Increased susceptibility to local infection
- Perioral dermatitis if used on face for prolonged period, although less common than w/ more potent corticosteroids

CORTICOSTEROIDS, TOPICAL, MID POTENCY

TRADE NAMES
(Generic in parentheses)
- Kenalog, Aristocort (triamcinolone)
- Valisone, Betatrex, Luxiq (betamethasone valerate)
- Cloderm (clocortolone)
- Cordran (flurandrenolide)
- Cutivate (fluticasone)
- Dermatop (prednicarbate)
- Synalar, Derma-Smoothe (fluocinolone)
- Elocon (mometasone)
- Locoid (hydrocortisone butyrate)
- Uticort (betamethasone benzoate)
- Diprosone, Maxivate, Alphatrex (betamethasone dipropionate)
- Westcort (hydrocortisone valerate)

GENERIC AVAILABLE
- Yes

DOSAGE FORM
- Cream
- Ointment
- Lotion
- Gel
- Foam

SIDE EFFECTS, COMMON OR MILD
- Dermatologic: skin atrophy, steroid addiction (rebound flare after discontinuing the medication), delayed wound healing, hypopigmentation, acneform eruption, striae

SIDE EFFECTS, SERIOUS
- Adrenal insufficiency (unusual)

DRUG INTERACTIONS
- None

PRECAUTIONS
- Tachyphylaxis if used more than twice daily for prolonged periods
- Increased susceptibility to local infection
- Perioral dermatitis if used on face for prolonged period

CORTICOSTEROIDS, TOPICAL, SUPER POTENCY

TRADE NAMES
(Generic in parentheses)
- Temovate, Ulux, Cormax, Embelline, Clobex (clobetasol)
- Ultravate (halobetasol)
- Diprolene AF (augmented betamethasone dipropionate)
- Psorcon, Maxiflor, Florone (diflorasone diacetate)
- Cordran (flurandrenolide tape)

GENERIC AVAILABLE
- Yes

DOSAGE FORM
- Cream
- Ointment
- Lotion
- Gel
- Foam
- Tape

SIDE EFFECTS, COMMON OR MILD
- Dermatologic: skin atrophy, steroid addition (rebound flare after discontinuing the medication), tachyphylaxis, increased

susceptibility to local infection, perioral dermatitis, delayed wound healing, hypopigmentation, acneform eruption, striae

SIDE EFFECTS, SERIOUS
- Adrenal suppression

DRUG INTERACTIONS
- None

PRECAUTIONS
- Apply for a maximum of 14 days w/out a 1-week rest period.
- Do not use on face.
- Apply in intertriginous areas for a maximum of 1 week.

CYCLOPHOSPHAMIDE

TRADE NAMES
- Cytoxan
- Neosar

GENERIC AVAILABLE
- No

DOSAGE FORM
- 25-mg, 50-mg tablets
- 100-mg, 200-mg, 300-mg vials for IV injection

SIDE EFFECTS, COMMON OR MILD
- Dermatologic: alopecia, stomatitis, dyspigmentation of skin & nails, skin eruption
- GI: nausea & vomiting, diarrhea
- GU: cystitis

SIDE EFFECTS, SERIOUS
- Dermatologic: anaphylaxis
- Cardiovascular: congestive failure, cardiomyopathy
- Bone marrow suppression
- GU: hemorrhagic cystitis, sterility; increased risk of bladder cancer

DRUG INTERACTIONS
- Bone marrow suppressants
- Allopurinol

- Doxorubicin
- Zidovudine

PRECAUTIONS
- Pts must drink large volumes of fluids to prevent interstitial cystitis.
- Use caution in pts w/ impaired renal or liver function, leukopenia or thrombocytopenia.

CYCLOSPORINE

TRADE NAMES
- Neoral
- Sandimmune
- SangCya

GENERIC AVAILABLE
- Yes

DOSAGE FORM
- Neoral: 25-mg, 100-mg capsule; 100 mg/mL oral solution
- Sandimmune: 25-mg, 50-mg, 100-mg capsule; 100 mg/mL oral solution; 50 mg/mL for IV infusion

SIDE EFFECTS, COMMON OR MILD
- Dermatologic: hypertrichosis, acne, gingival hyperplasia
- GI: nausea & vomiting, diarrhea, abdominal pain

SIDE EFFECTS, SERIOUS
- Dermatologic: anaphylaxis
- Bone marrow suppression
- Renal: nephrotoxicity
- Neurologic: seizures

DRUG INTERACTIONS
- Antifungal agents
- Anticonvulsants
- Carboplatin
- Cimetidine
- Ciprofloxacin
- Colchicine
- Oral contraceptives

- Diltiazem
- Erythromycin
- Statins
- Glyburide/metformin
- Metronidazole
- Nafcillin
- Nonsteroidal anti-inflammatory agents
- Pimozide
- Protease inhibitors
- Rifampin
- Verapamil
- Vinca alkaloids

PRECAUTIONS
- Grapefruit juice ingestion may increase blood levels of the drug.
- Use caution in pts w/ impaired renal or hepatic function & those taking other potentially nephrotoxic drugs.
- Decreased magnesium levels w/ prolonged use.

DAPSONE

TRADE NAMES
- None

GENERIC AVAILABLE
- Yes

DOSAGE FORM
- 25-mg, 100-mg tablet

SIDE EFFECTS, COMMON OR MILD
- Dermatologic: skin eruption, including urticaria; photosensitivity
- GI: nausea & vomiting, abdominal pain
- General: malaise
- Neurologic: dizziness, peripheral neuropathy

SIDE EFFECTS, SERIOUS
- Dermatologic: dapsone hypersensitivity syndrome, exfoliative dermatitis, toxic epidermal necrolysis

- Hematologic: agranulocytosis, leukopenia, methemoglobinemia, hemolytic anemia if G6PD deficient
- Renal: acute tubular necrosis
- GI: hepatotoxicity, pancreatitis

DRUG INTERACTIONS
- Antacids
- Bone marrow suppressants
- Clozapine
- Cytotoxic chemotherapeutic agents
- Interferon
- Probenecid
- Trimethoprim
- Zidovudine

PRECAUTIONS
- Increased hemolysis in pts w/ G-6PD deficiency.

DICLOXACILLIN

TRADE NAMES
- Dynapen

GENERIC AVAILABLE
- Yes

DOSAGE FORM
- 250-mg, 500-mg tablet

SIDE EFFECTS, COMMON OR MILD
- Dermatologic: urticaria & other vascular reactions
- GI: nausea & vomiting, diarrhea

SIDE EFFECTS, SERIOUS
- Dermatologic: anaphylaxis, Stevens-Johnson syndrome, toxic epidermal necrolysis
- GI: pseudomembranous colitis
- Bone marrow: thrombocytopenia
- Renal: interstitial nephritis

DRUG INTERACTIONS

- Aminoglycoside antibiotics
- Oral contraceptives
- Methotrexate
- Probenecid

PRECAUTIONS

- Use w/ caution in pts w/ cephalosporin allergy, seizure disorder or impaired renal function.

DOXYCYCLINE

TRADE NAMES

- Vibramycin
- Doryx
- Vibra-Tabs
- Monodox
- Periostat

GENERIC AVAILABLE

- Yes

DOSAGE FORM

- 20-mg, 50-mg, 100-mg tablet

SIDE EFFECTS, COMMON OR MILD

- Dermatologic: photosensitivity, stomatitis, oral candidiasis, urticaria or other vascular reaction
- GI: nausea & vomiting, diarrhea, esophagitis
- Neurologic: tinnitus, dizziness, drowsiness, headache, ataxia

SIDE EFFECTS, SERIOUS

- GI: pseudomembranous colitis, hepatotoxicity
- Neurologic: pseudotumor cerebri
- Hematologic: neutropenia, thrombocytopenia

DRUG INTERACTIONS

- Antacids
- Calcium, magnesium or iron salts
- Oral contraceptives
- Digoxin

- Isotretinoin
- Warfarin

PRECAUTIONS
- Contraindicated in pts <8 years old.

EFLORNITHINE

TRADE NAMES
- Vaniqa

GENERIC AVAILABLE
- No

DOSAGE FORM
- 13.9% cream

SIDE EFFECTS, COMMON OR MILD
- Dermatologic: stinging, burning sensation, irritant contact dermatitis, acneform eruption, pseudofolliculitis barbae

SIDE EFFECTS, SERIOUS
- None

DRUG INTERACTIONS
- None

PRECAUTIONS
- Slows hair regrowth, but does not cause permanent hair loss.

ERYTHROMYCIN, SYSTEMIC

TRADE NAMES
- Eryc
- E-mycin
- PCE
- EES
- Ilosone

GENERIC AVAILABLE
- Yes

DOSAGE FORM
- 250-mg, 333-mg, 400-mg, 500-mg tablet
- 200 mg/5 mL, 400 mg/5 mL suspension

SIDE EFFECTS, COMMON OR MILD
- Dermatologic: urticaria or other vascular reaction, stomatitis
- GI: nausea & vomiting, diarrhea, abdominal cramps, jaundice

SIDE EFFECTS, SERIOUS
- Dermatologic: anaphylaxis, Stevens-Johnson syndrome
- Bone marrow suppression
- Cardiovascular: arrhythmias, hypotension

DRUG INTERACTIONS
- Amiodarone
- Amitriptyline
- Budesonide
- Buspirone
- Carbamazepine
- Clozapine
- Oral contraceptives
- Cyclosporine
- Digoxin
- Ergot alkaloids
- Methadone
- Phenytoin
- Pimozide
- Protease inhibitors
- Quinidine
- Statins
- Tacrolimus
- Theophylline
- Valproic acid
- Vinca alkaloids
- Warfarin

PRECAUTIONS
- Use caution in pts w/ myasthenia gravis or impaired liver function.

ERYTHROMYCIN, TOPICAL

TRADE NAMES
- Emgel
- Erycette
- EryDerm
- Erymax
- Erythra-Derm
- T-Stat
- Theramycin
- Staticin

GENERIC AVAILABLE
- Yes

DOSAGE FORM
- 2% gel
- 1.5%, 2% solution

SIDE EFFECTS, COMMON OR MILD
- Dermatologic: burning sensation, dryness, peeling, pruritus, erythema

SIDE EFFECTS, SERIOUS
- None

DRUG INTERACTIONS
- Topical clindamycin

PRECAUTIONS
- High rate of bacterial resistance if used alone; decreased rate of bacterial resistance if used w/ benzoyl peroxide

FINASTERIDE

TRADE NAMES
- Propecia

GENERIC AVAILABLE
- No

DOSAGE FORM
- 1-mg tablet

SIDE EFFECTS, COMMON OR MILD
- GU: decreased libido, impotence, decreased ejaculate volume

SIDE EFFECTS, SERIOUS
- None

DRUG INTERACTIONS
- None

PRECAUTIONS
- May take 4–6 months to see effects of therapy.

FLUCONAZOLE

TRADE NAMES
- Diflucan

GENERIC AVAILABLE
- No

DOSAGE FORM
- 50-mg, 100-mg, 150-mg, 200-mg tablet
- 50 mg/mL, 200 mg/mL suspension

SIDE EFFECTS, COMMON OR MILD
- Dermatologic: skin eruption
- GI: nausea & vomiting, diarrhea, abdominal pain, dyspepsia
- Neurologic: headache, dizziness, taste changes

SIDE EFFECTS, SERIOUS
- Dermatologic: angioedema, Stevens-Johnson syndrome
- GI: hepatotoxicity
- Neurologic: seizures
- Hematologic: agranulocytosis

DRUG INTERACTIONS
- Amitriptyline
- Barbiturates
- Buspirone

- Carbamazepine
- Celecoxib
- Cyclosporine
- Digoxin
- Ergot alkaloids
- Glyburide/metformin
- Phenytoin
- Pimozide
- Protease inhibitors
- Quinidine
- Rifampin
- Statins
- Sulfonylureas
- Tacrolimus
- Theophyllines
- Warfarin

PRECAUTIONS
- Use caution in pts w/ impaired renal or hepatic function.

FLUOROURACIL, TOPICAL

TRADE NAMES
- Efudex
- Fluoroplex
- Carac

GENERIC AVAILABLE
- No

DOSAGE FORM
- 0.5%, 1%, 5% cream
- 1%, 2% solution

SIDE EFFECTS, COMMON OR MILD
- Dermatologic: local pain, pruritus, burning, crusting, erosions, allergic contact dermatitis, photosensitivity, dyspigmentation

SIDE EFFECTS, SERIOUS
- None

DRUG INTERACTIONS
- None

PRECAUTIONS
- Signs of inflammation may last for weeks after discontinuing therapy.

GRISEOFULVIN

TRADE NAMES
- Fulvicin P/G
- Gris-PEG
- Grifulvin V

GENERIC AVAILABLE
- Yes

DOSAGE FORM
- 125-mg, 165-mg, 250-mg, 330-mg tablet
- 125 mg/5 mL suspension

SIDE EFFECTS, COMMON OR MILD
- Skin: photosensitivity, vascular reaction
- GI: nausea & vomiting, diarrhea, flatulence
- Neurologic: dizziness, paresthesias, confusion

SIDE EFFECTS, SERIOUS
- GI: hepatotoxicity
- Bone marrow: granulocytopenia

DRUG INTERACTIONS
- Amiodarone
- Barbiturates
- Carbamazepine
- Clarithromycin
- Oral contraceptives
- Cyclosporine
- Erythromycin
- Itraconazole
- Ketoconazole
- Protease inhibitors

- Tacrolimus
- Warfarin

PRECAUTIONS
- Contraindicated in pts w/ acute intermittent porphyria or during pregnancy.
- Use caution in pts w/ penicillin allergy or impaired liver function.

HYDROQUINONE

TRADE NAMES
- Solaquin Forte
- Eldoquin
- Eldopaque
- Nuquin
- Lustra
- Melanex
- Esoterica
- Porcelana Fade Cream
- Epi-Quin Micro
- Tri-Luma

GENERIC AVAILABLE
- Yes

DOSAGE FORM
- 1.5% cream (Eldopaque, Esoterica, Porcelana)
- 2% cream (Nuquin)
- 3% lotion (Melanex)
- 4% cream (Solaquin Forte, Lustra)
- 4% gel (Solaquin Forte)
- 4% cream w/ tretinoin & fluocinolone (Tri-Luma)

SIDE EFFECTS, COMMON OR MILD
- Dermatologic: contact dermatitis, burning sensation, erythema

SIDE EFFECTS, SERIOUS
- Ochronosis-like pigmentation

DRUG INTERACTIONS
- None

PRECAUTIONS
- It may take several months to see positive results of therapy.

HYDROXYCHLOROQUINE

TRADE NAMES
- Plaquenil

GENERIC AVAILABLE
- Yes

DOSAGE FORM
- 200-mg tablet

SIDE EFFECTS, COMMON OR MILD
- Dermatologic: blue-gray skin discoloration, transverse nail bands, skin eruptions
- GI: nausea & vomiting, diarrhea
- Ocular: halos, blurred vision
- Neurologic: headache, nervousness, mood swings, vertigo

SIDE EFFECTS, SERIOUS
- Ocular: visual changes from retinopathy
- Hematologic: agranulocytosis, aplastic anemia
- Neurologic: seizures

DRUG INTERACTIONS
- None

PRECAUTIONS
- May exacerbate psoriasis.
- May produce asymptomatic liver enzyme elevation.
    - ➤ Decreased efficacy in smokers

HYDROXYUREA

TRADE NAMES
- Hydrea

GENERIC AVAILABLE
- Yes

DOSAGE FORM
- 500-mg tablet

SIDE EFFECTS, COMMON OR MILD
- Dermatologic: stomatitis, alopecia, erythema, skin eruption, painful leg ulcers
- GI: hepatitis, anorexia, nausea & vomiting, diarrhea, dyspepsia
- Neurologic: headache, dizziness, hallucinations, seizures

SIDE EFFECTS, SERIOUS
- Pulmonary: pulmonary fibrosis
- Bone marrow: anemia, thrombocytopenia, leukopenia
- Renal: renal insufficiency

DRUG INTERACTIONS
- Other bone marrow suppressive agents

PRECAUTIONS
- Use caution in pts w/ impaired renal function.
- May predispose pt to leukemia.

IMIQUIMOD

TRADE NAMES
- Aldara

GENERIC AVAILABLE
- No

DOSAGE FORM
- 5% cream

SIDE EFFECTS, COMMON OR MILD
- Dermatologic: burning sensation, irritant dermatitis, pruritus, local pain, hypopigmentation

SIDE EFFECTS, SERIOUS
- None

DRUG INTERACTIONS
- None

PRECAUTIONS
- None

ISOTRETINOIN

TRADE NAMES
- Accutane
- Amnesteem
- Sotret
- Claravis

GENERIC AVAILABLE
- Yes

DOSAGE FORM
- 10-mg, 20-mg, 30-mg, 40-mg capsule

SIDE EFFECTS, COMMON OR MILD
- Dermatologic: peeling on hands & feet, cheilitis, skin fragility, alopecia, dry skin, pruritus, paronychia
- Eyes: dry eyes, w/ contact lens intolerance; dry mucous membranes
- Musculoskeletal: myalgias, arthralgias, spinal hyperostosis

SIDE EFFECTS, SERIOUS
- Eye: decreased night vision
- Neurologic: pseudotumor cerebri; mood disorder, particularly depression
- GI: hepatotoxicity, pancreatitis
- GU: major birth defects

DRUG INTERACTIONS
- Tretinoin
- Benzoyl peroxide
- Carbamazepine
- Tetracycline

PRECAUTIONS

- Pregnancy is absolute contraindication.
- Hyperlipidemia, w/ rare pancreatitis, particularly in pts w/ pre-existent high serum lipids
- Must be prescribed through iPledge program

ITRACONAZOLE

TRADE NAMES

- Sporanox

GENERIC AVAILABLE

- No

DOSAGE FORM

- 100-mg tablet
- 10 mg/mL oral solution

SIDE EFFECTS, COMMON OR MILD

- Dermatologic: skin eruption, vasculitis
- GI: nausea & vomiting, diarrhea, dyspepsia

SIDE EFFECTS, SERIOUS

- Dermatologic: anaphylaxis, Stevens-Johnson syndrome reaction
- GI: hepatotoxicity

DRUG INTERACTIONS

- Amiodarone
- Amitriptyline
- Antacids
- Anticonvulsants
- Buspirone
- Cyclosporine
- Digoxin
- Glyburide/metformin
- Protease inhibitors
- Pimozide
- Quinidine
- Rifampin
- Statins

- Sulfonylureas
- Theophylline
- Vinca alkaloids
- Warfarin

PRECAUTIONS
- Use caution in pts w/ cardiovascular or pulmonary disease, impaired liver or renal function.
- Pt may develop elevated liver enzymes and/or hypertriglyceridemia.

IVERMECTIN

TRADE NAMES
- Stromectol

GENERIC AVAILABLE
- Yes

DOSAGE FORM
- 3-mg, 6-mg tablet

SIDE EFFECTS, COMMON OR MILD
- Dermatologic: pruritus, skin eruption, edema
- Lymph nodes: lymphadenopathy
- Neurologic: dizziness

SIDE EFFECTS, SERIOUS
- None

DRUG INTERACTIONS
- None

PRECAUTIONS
- None

KETOCONAZOLE

TRADE NAMES
- Nizoral

GENERIC AVAILABLE
- Yes

DOSAGE FORM
- 200-mg tablet

SIDE EFFECTS, COMMON OR MILD
- Dermatologic: skin eruption, pruritus
- GI: nausea & vomiting, diarrhea, abdominal pain
- Neurologic: somnolence, dizziness, lethargy, headache, nervousness

SIDE EFFECTS, SERIOUS
- Dermatologic: anaphylaxis
- GI: hepatic failure
- Endocrine: adrenal insufficiency

DRUG INTERACTIONS
- Amitriptyline
- Anticonvulsants
- Buspirone
- Celecoxib
- Cyclosporine
- Digoxin
- Ergot alkaloids
- Glyburide/metformin
- Pimozide
- Protease inhibitors
- Quinidine
- Rifampin
- Statins
- Sulfonylureas
- Theophylline
- Warfarin

PRECAUTIONS
- Use caution in pts w/ hepatic insufficiency.
- Poor gastric absorption in pts w/ achlorhydria.

LINDANE

TRADE NAMES
- None

GENERIC AVAILABLE
- Yes

DOSAGE FORM
- 1% lotion
- 1% shampoo

SIDE EFFECTS, COMMON OR MILD
- Skin: irritant dermatitis
- Neurologic: dizziness, anxiety, CNS stimulation

SIDE EFFECTS, SERIOUS
- Neurologic: seizures

DRUG INTERACTIONS
- None

PRECAUTIONS
- Contraindicated in pregnancy; lactation; crusted scabies; or children <2 years old.

METHOTREXATE

TRADE NAMES
- Rheumatrex

GENERIC AVAILABLE
- Yes

DOSAGE FORM
- 2.5-mg tablet
- 25 mg/mL solution for intramuscular injection

SIDE EFFECTS, COMMON OR MILD
- Dermatologic: stomatitis, photosensitivity, skin eruption, alopecia

- GI: nausea, vomiting
- General: fatigue

SIDE EFFECTS, SERIOUS
- Dermatologic: Stevens-Johnson syndrome, toxic epidermal necrolysis, exfoliative dermatitis, radiation recall reaction
- Pulmonary: pulmonary fibrosis
- Bone marrow suppression

DRUG INTERACTIONS
- Acitretin
- COX-2 inhibitors
- Salicylates & other nonsteroidal anti-inflammatory agents
- Penicillins
- Sulfonamides, especially Bactrim or Septra
- Trimethoprim

PRECAUTIONS
- Contraindicated in pregnant pts & pts w/ alcohol abuse, severe liver dysfunction & immunodeficiency syndromes.
- Use caution in pts w/ impaired renal function or ulcerative colitis.

METHOXSALEN

TRADE NAMES
- Oxsoralen Ultra
- Oxsoralen lotion

GENERIC AVAILABLE
- No

DOSAGE FORM
- 10-mg capsule
- 1% solution for dilution

SIDE EFFECTS, COMMON OR MILD
- Skin: phototoxic reaction, exanthem, herpes simplex virus infection recurrence, photo-aging after chronic use
- GI: nausea, vomiting, hepatic toxicity

SIDE EFFECTS, SERIOUS
- Skin: increased risk for skin cancer, particularly squamous cell carcinoma
- Ocular: cataract formation

DRUG INTERACTIONS
- Doxycycline & other photosensitizers
- Fluoroquinolones
- Carbamazepine
- Phenytoin

PRECAUTIONS
- Strict sun avoidance on day of oral administration.

METRONIDAZOLE, TOPICAL

TRADE NAMES
- MetroGel
- MetroCream
- MetroLotion
- Noritate
- Rozex

GENERIC AVAILABLE
- Yes

DOSAGE FORM
- 0.75% cream, gel, emulsion
- 1% cream

SIDE EFFECTS, COMMON OR MILD
- Dermatologic: burning sensation, erythema, skin eruption

SIDE EFFECTS, SERIOUS
- None

DRUG INTERACTIONS
- None

PRECAUTIONS
- None

MINOCYCLINE

TRADE NAMES
- Minocin
- Dynacin
- Vectrin

GENERIC AVAILABLE
- Yes

DOSAGE FORM
- 50-mg, 75-mg, 100-mg tablet

SIDE EFFECTS, COMMON OR MILD
- Dermatologic: photosensitivity, stomatitis, oral candidiasis, urticaria or other vascular reaction
- GI: nausea & vomiting, diarrhea, esophagitis
- Neurologic: tinnitus, dizziness, drowsiness, headache, ataxia

SIDE EFFECTS, SERIOUS
- GI: pseudomembranous colitis, hepatotoxicity
- Neurologic: pseudotumor cerebri
- Hematologic: neutropenia, thrombocytopenia

DRUG INTERACTIONS
- Antacids
- Calcium, magnesium or iron salts
- Oral contraceptives
- Digoxin
- Isotretinoin
- Warfarin

PRECAUTIONS
- Contraindicated in pregnancy & in pts <8 years old.
- Use caution in pts w/ impaired renal or liver function.

MINOXIDIL, TOPICAL

TRADE NAMES
- Rogaine

GENERIC AVAILABLE
- Yes

DOSAGE FORM
- 2%, 5% solution

SIDE EFFECTS, COMMON OR MILD
- Dermatologic: irritant dermatitis, hypertrichosis

SIDE EFFECTS, SERIOUS
- None

DRUG INTERACTIONS
- None

PRECAUTIONS
- May take up to 6 months to see effects

MUPIROCIN

TRADE NAMES
- Bactroban
- Centany

GENERIC AVAILABLE
- Yes

DOSAGE FORM
- 2% cream, ointment

SIDE EFFECTS, COMMON OR MILD
- Dermatologic: burning sensation, dryness, pruritus, redness

SIDE EFFECTS, SERIOUS
- Superinfection after prolonged use

DRUG INTERACTIONS
- None

PRECAUTIONS
- Use caution when applying to large open wounds.

MYCOPHENOLATE MOFETIL

TRADE NAMES
- CellCept

GENERIC AVAILABLE
- No

DOSAGE FORM
- 250-mg, 500-mg tablet

SIDE EFFECTS, COMMON OR MILD
- GI: diarrhea, abdominal pain, nausea & vomiting
- Neurologic: headache
- Cardiovascular: peripheral edema
- Pulmonary: cough
- GU: urinary urgency, frequency & dysuria
- Hematologic: leukopenia

SIDE EFFECTS, SERIOUS
- Hematologic: bone marrow suppression, immunosuppression
- Infectious: increased susceptibility to infection
- GI: bleeding, ulceration, bowel perforation

DRUG INTERACTIONS
- Acyclovir
- Azathioprine
- Oral contraceptives
- Ganciclovir
- Iron salts
- Probenecid

PRECAUTIONS
- Use caution in pts w/ severe renal or GI disease or bone marrow suppression.
- Pt may develop hypokalemia, hypercholesterolemia.
- May predispose to malignancy.

NAFTIFINE

TRADE NAMES
- Naftin

GENERIC AVAILABLE
- No

DOSAGE FORM
- 1% cream
- 1% gel

SIDE EFFECTS, COMMON OR MILD
- Dermatologic: burning sensation, pruritus, erythema, dryness

SIDE EFFECTS, SERIOUS
- None

DRUG INTERACTIONS
- None

PRECAUTIONS
- None

NIACINAMIDE

TRADE NAMES
- None

GENERIC AVAILABLE
- Yes

DOSAGE FORM
- 500-mg tablet

SIDE EFFECTS, COMMON OR MILD
- GI: dyspepsia
- Neurologic: headache

SIDE EFFECTS, SERIOUS
- GI: hepatic toxicity

DRUG INTERACTIONS
- None

PRECAUTIONS
- None

PENICILLIN G BENZATHINE

TRADE NAMES
- Bicillin LA

GENERIC AVAILABLE
- Yes

DOSAGE FORM
- 300,000 units/mL; 600,000 units/mL for intramuscular injection

SIDE EFFECTS, COMMON OR MILD
- Dermatologic: urticaria & other skin eruptions
- GI: nausea & vomiting, diarrhea

SIDE EFFECTS, SERIOUS
- Dermatologic: anaphylaxis
- Bone marrow: thrombocytopenia
- GI: pseudomembranous colitis
- Renal: interstitial nephritis

DRUG INTERACTIONS
- Aminoglycoside antibiotics
- Oral contraceptives
- Methotrexate
- Probenecid

PRECAUTIONS
- Use caution in pts w/ cephalosporin allergy, seizure disorder or impaired renal function.

PENICILLIN VK

TRADE NAMES
- Pen-Vee K
- Veetids

GENERIC AVAILABLE
- Yes

DOSAGE FORM
- 250-mg, 500-mg tablet
- 125 mg/5 mL, 250 mg/mL suspension

SIDE EFFECTS, COMMON OR MILD
- Dermatologic: urticaria & other skin eruptions
- GI: nausea & vomiting, diarrhea

SIDE EFFECTS, SERIOUS
- Dermatologic: anaphylaxis, Stevens-Johnson syndrome, toxic epidermal necrolysis
- GI: pseudomembranous colitis
- Renal: interstitial nephritis
- Bone marrow: thrombocytopenia

DRUG INTERACTIONS
- Aminoglycoside antibiotics
- Oral contraceptives
- Methotrexate
- Probenecid

PRECAUTIONS
- Use caution in pts w/ cephalosporin allergy, seizure disorder or impaired renal function.

PERMETHRIN

TRADE NAMES
- Elimite
- Nix

GENERIC AVAILABLE
- No

DOSAGE FORM
- 5% cream
- 1% cream rinse

SIDE EFFECTS, COMMON OR MILD
- Dermatologic: pruritus, redness, scalp swelling

SIDE EFFECTS, SERIOUS
- None

DRUG INTERACTIONS
- None

PRECAUTIONS
- None

PODOFILOX

TRADE NAMES
- Condylox

GENERIC AVAILABLE
- No

DOSAGE FORM
- 0.5% solution
- 0.5% gel

SIDE EFFECTS, COMMON OR MILD
- Dermatologic: burning sensation, irritant dermatitis

SIDE EFFECTS, SERIOUS
- None

DRUG INTERACTIONS
- None

PRECAUTIONS
- Limited usefulness on non-mucous membrane skin.

PREDNISONE

TRADE NAMES
- Deltasone
- Sterapred

GENERIC AVAILABLE
- Yes

DOSAGE FORM
- 1-mg, 2.5-mg, 5-mg, 10-mg, 20-mg, 50-mg tablet

SIDE EFFECTS, COMMON OR MILD
- Dermatologic: skin fragility & ecchymoses, skin atrophy, impaired wound healing
- GI: nausea, vomiting, dyspepsia, weight gain
- GU: menstrual irregularities
- Endocrine: cushingoid features, hyperglycemia
- Cardiovascular: hypertension, fluid retention
- Musculoskeletal: osteopenia
- Neurologic: mood change, insomnia

SIDE EFFECTS, SERIOUS
- GI: peptic ulcer
- GU: menstrual irregularities
- Endocrine: adrenal insufficiency upon withdrawal
- Cardiovascular: congestive heart failure
- Infectious: increased susceptibility to infection
- Musculoskeletal: aseptic hip necrosis
- Neurologic: psychosis, pseudotumor cerebri

DRUG INTERACTIONS
- Barbiturates
- Phenytoin
- Beta agonists
- COX-2 inhibitors
- Cyclosporine
- Digoxin
- Thiazide diuretics
- Glyburide/metformin
- Nonsteroidal anti-inflammatory agents
- Rifampin
- Warfarin
- Many others

PRECAUTIONS
- Contraindicated in pts w/ systemic fungal infections.

- Use caution in pts w/ congestive heart failure, seizure disorder, hypertension, diabetes mellitus, tuberculosis, osteoporosis or impaired hepatic function.

RIFAMPIN

TRADE NAMES
- Rifadin
- Rimactane

GENERIC AVAILABLE
- Yes

DOSAGE FORM
- 150-mg, 300-mg capsule

SIDE EFFECTS, COMMON OR MILD
- Dermatologic: pruritus, urticaria or other eruptions
- GI: abdominal pain, nausea & vomiting, diarrhea
- Neurologic: dizziness, ataxia, headache

SIDE EFFECTS, SERIOUS
- Renal: renal failure, interstitial nephritis
- GI: hepatotoxicity
- Bone marrow: thrombocytopenia, leukopenia

DRUG INTERACTIONS
- Digoxin
- Chloramphenicol
- Warfarin
- Phenobarbital
- Phenytoin
- Ketoconazole
- Theophylline
- Verapamil
- Cyclosporine
- Systemic corticosteroids
- Oral contraceptives
- Dapsone
- Sulfonylureas

PRECAUTIONS
- Pt may develop red-colored secretions (eg, tears).
- May stain contact lenses.
- Pt may develop asymptomatic liver enzyme elevation.

SELECTIVE SEROTONIN REUPTAKE INHIBITORS

TRADE NAMES
(Generic names in parentheses)
- Celexa (citalopram)
- Zoloft (sertraline)
- Prozac (fluoxetine)
- Paxil (paroxetine)
- Luvox (fluvoxamine)

GENERIC AVAILABLE
- Yes

DOSAGE FORM
- Celexa: 20-mg, 40-mg tablet
- Zoloft: 25-mg, 50-mg, 100-mg tablet
- Prozac: 10-mg, 20-mg tablet; 20 mg/5 mL liquid
- Paxil: 20-mg, 30-mg tablet
- Luvox: 25-mg, 50-mg, 100-mg tablet

SIDE EFFECTS, COMMON OR MILD
- Dermatologic: skin eruption
- GI: anorexia, increased appetite
- Neurologic: insomnia, sedation, headache
- GU: sexual dysfunction

SIDE EFFECTS, SERIOUS
- Serotonin syndrome

DRUG INTERACTIONS
- Cimetidine
- Ergot alkaloids
- Ethanol
- Other psychotropic drugs, including atypical & typical antipsychotic agents, lithium, MAO inhibitors, tricyclics & buspirone

- Metoprolol
- Phenytoin
- Quinidine
- Warfarin

PRECAUTIONS
- Do not start within 14 days of MAO inhibitor use.
- Avoid rapid withdrawal.

SPIRONOLACTONE

TRADE NAMES
- Aldactone

GENERIC AVAILABLE
- Yes

DOSAGE FORM
- 25-mg, 50-mg, 100-mg tablet

SIDE EFFECTS, COMMON OR MILD
- Dermatologic: skin eruption
- GI: dyspepsia
- Neurologic: sedation, headache
- GU: sexual dysfunction, dysmenorrhea

SIDE EFFECTS, SERIOUS
- Dermatologic: anaphylaxis
- Bone marrow suppression

DRUG INTERACTIONS
- ACE inhibitors
- Cyclosporine
- Nonsteroidal anti-inflammatory agents
- COX-2 inhibitors
- Potassium salts
- Tacrolimus

PRECAUTIONS
- Contraindicated in pts w/ renal insufficiency, hyperkalemia.
- Use caution in pts w/ hepatic dysfunction.

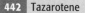

TAZAROTENE

TRADE NAMES
- Tazorac

GENERIC AVAILABLE
- No

DOSAGE FORM
- 0.05%, 0.1% gel

SIDE EFFECTS, COMMON OR MILD
- Dermatologic: irritant dermatitis, photosensitivity

SIDE EFFECTS, SERIOUS
- None

DRUG INTERACTIONS
- Benzoyl peroxide
- Isotretinoin
- Photosensitizing drugs

PRECAUTIONS
- Avoid applying near the eye.

TERBINAFINE

TRADE NAMES
- Lamisil

GENERIC AVAILABLE
- No

DOSAGE FORM
- 250-mg tablet
- 1% cream

SIDE EFFECTS, COMMON OR MILD
- Topical formulation
  - Dermatologic: irritant dermatitis
- Oral formulation
  - Dermatologic: skin eruption, pruritus
  - GI: nausea & vomiting, diarrhea, dyspepsia
  - Neurologic: taste changes

SIDE EFFECTS, SERIOUS
- Topical formulation: none
- Oral formulation
  - ➤ Dermatologic: Stevens-Johnson syndrome, toxic epidermal necrolysis, anaphylaxis
  - ➤ GI: hepatotoxicity

DRUG INTERACTIONS
- Cimetidine
- Cyclosporine
- Rifampin
- Theophylline
- Thioridazine
- Tricyclic antidepressants

PRECAUTIONS
- Pt may develop asymptomatic liver enzyme elevation.
- Use caution in pts w/ impaired liver or renal function.

TETRACYCLINE

TRADE NAMES
- Sumycin

GENERIC AVAILABLE
- Yes

DOSAGE FORM
- 250-mg, 500-mg capsule

SIDE EFFECTS, COMMON OR MILD
- Dermatologic: photosensitivity, stomatitis, oral candidiasis, urticaria or other vascular reaction
- GI: nausea & vomiting, diarrhea, esophagitis
- Neurologic: tinnitus, dizziness, drowsiness, headache, ataxia

SIDE EFFECTS, SERIOUS
- GI: pseudomembranous colitis, hepatotoxicity
- Neurologic: pseudotumor cerebri
- Hematologic: neutropenia, thrombocytopenia

DRUG INTERACTIONS
- Antacids
- Calcium, magnesium or iron salts
- Oral contraceptives
- Digoxin
- Isotretinoin
- Warfarin

PRECAUTIONS
- Contraindicated in pregnancy or in pts <8 years old.
- Use caution in pts w/ impaired renal or hepatic function.

THALIDOMIDE

TRADE NAMES
- Thalomid

GENERIC AVAILABLE
- No

DOSAGE FORM
- 50-mg, 100-mg, 200-mg tablet

SIDE EFFECTS, COMMON OR MILD
- Skin: eruption, photosensitivity
- GI: increased appetite & weight gain, diarrhea
- Constitutional: fever, chills
- Neurologic: somnolence, mood changes, confusion, amnesia, headache

SIDE EFFECTS, SERIOUS
- Skin: Stevens-Johnson syndrome, toxic epidermal necrolysis
- Neurologic: peripheral neuropathy, seizures
- Pregnancy: severe birth defects
- Cardiovascular: severe hypertension, bradycardia
- Bone marrow: neutropenia

DRUG INTERACTIONS
- Acetaminophen
- Antihistamines
- Antipsychotics

- Anticonvulsants
- Protease inhibitors
- Griseofulvin
- Rifampin
- Opiates
- Sedative-hypnotics

PRECAUTIONS
- Contraindicated in pregnancy or in pts w/ moderate to severe pre-existing peripheral neuropathy.
- Use caution in pts w/ seizure disorder, cardiovascular disease or child-bearing potential.

THIOGUANINE

TRADE NAMES
- Thioguanine

GENERIC AVAILABLE
- No

DOSAGE FORM
- 40-mg tablet

SIDE EFFECTS, COMMON OR MILD
- GI: diarrhea, nausea, vomiting
- Neurologic: headache, fatigue

SIDE EFFECTS, SERIOUS
- GI: hepatotoxicity
- Bone marrow: myelosuppression

DRUG INTERACTIONS
- Azathioprine
- Sulfasalazine
- Busulfan

PRECAUTIONS
- Use caution in pts w/ low level of thiopurine methyltransferase.

TRETINOIN

TRADE NAMES
- Retin-A
- Retin-A Micro
- Avita
- Renova

GENERIC AVAILABLE
- Yes

DOSAGE FORM
- 0.025% cream
- 0.025% gel
- 0.05% cream
- 0.1% cream
- 0.04% micro gel
- 0.1% micro gel

SIDE EFFECTS, COMMON OR MILD
- Dermatologic: irritant dermatitis, photosensitivity

SIDE EFFECTS, SERIOUS
- None

DRUG INTERACTIONS
- Benzoyl peroxide
- Isotretinoin
- Photosensitizing drugs

PRECAUTIONS
- Avoid application near the eye.

VALACYCLOVIR

TRADE NAMES
- Valtrex

GENERIC AVAILABLE
- No

DOSAGE FORM
- 500-mg, 1,000-mg tablet

SIDE EFFECTS, COMMON OR MILD
- GI: nausea & vomiting
- Neurologic: headache

SIDE EFFECTS, SERIOUS
- GI: hepatitis
- Neurologic: seizures, encephalopathy, coma
- Bone marrow suppression

DRUG INTERACTIONS
- Aminoglycoside antibiotics
- Carboplatin
- Cidofovir
- Cisplatin
- Glyburide
- Metformin
- Mycophenolate mofetil
- Probenecid
- Nephrotoxic agents

PRECAUTIONS
- Use caution in elderly pts or those w/ renal insufficiency.